Hormones and Metabolic Control

A medical student's guide to control of various aspects of normal and abnormal metabolism

Second edition

DAVID A. WHITE BSc, PhD

Senior Lecturer, Department of Biochemistry,
University of Nottingham Medical School,
Nottingham, UK

and

MICHAEL BAXTER PhD, MRCP

Consultant Endocrinologist,
St Peter's Hospital, Chertsey, Surrey, UK

Edward Arnold
A member of the Hodder Headline Group
LONDON BOSTON MELBOURNE AUCKLAND

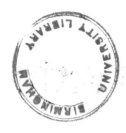

© 1994 David A White and Michael Baxter

First published in Great Britain 1984
Second edition 1994.

Distributed in the Americas by Little, Brown and Company
34 Beacon Street, Boston, MA 02108

British Library Cataloguing in Publication Data

White, David A.
   Hormones and Metabolic Control: Medical
   Student's Guide to Control of Various
   Aspects of Normal and Abnormal
   Metabolism. – 2Rev. ed
   I. Title
   612.39

ISBN 0–340–56355–9

1733522

Whilst the advice and information in this book is believed to be true
and accurate at the date of going to press, neither the authors nor
the publisher can accept any legal responsibility or liability for any
errors or omissions that may be made. In particular (but without
limiting the generality of the preceding disclaimer) every effort
has been made to check drug dosages; however, it is still possible
that errors have been missed. Furthermore, dosage schedules are
constantly being revised and new side effects recognised. For these
reasons the reader is strongly urged to consult the drug companies'
printed instructions before administering any of the drugs
recommended in this book.

Typeset in Baskerville by Anneset, Weston-super-Mare, Avon.
Printed in Great Britain for Edward Arnold, a division of
Hodder Headline PLC, Mill Road, Dunton Green, Sevenoaks,
Kent TN13 2YA by St. Edmundsbury Press Ltd., Bury St.
Edmunds, Suffolk and bound by Hunter & Foulis Ltd, Edinburgh.

Preface

The expansion in knowledge and understanding in the basic medical sciences presents a difficult dilemma for those involved in the teaching of medical students – what should be included in the curriculum and in what detail should it be taught? Can the principles be taught without the fine print? In preparing this second edition we have been cognisant of the overloading of the present curriculum and of the recent discussion paper on undergraduate medical teaching from the General Medical Council. One of the educational aims proposed in that paper 'is to develop an attitude to learning that is based on curiosity and the exploration of knowledge rather than on its passive acquisition'. It also suggests that basic medical sciences be extended through the entire medical course rather than restricted to the first two years.

We had such ideas in mind in the first edition where we sought to put basic metabolism into context in man and tried to illustrate how a knowledge of metabolic pathways and their control might help in understanding normal homoeostasis and abnormal metabolic states. This approach proved successful with our own students in Nottingham where ordered and disordered metabolism courses are popular and do not attract the bad press that basic biochemistry and metabolic pathways traditionally receive from the preclinical student consumer.

As in the first edition, the current text assumes that the reader has access to standard textbooks of biochemistry and physiology although it may be argued that detailed knowledge of individual metabolic pathways, other than points of control, is not crucial to an understanding of the importance of the overall processes. It was with great reluctance that structural formulae have been included, albeit in only one chapter, but hormone biosynthesis was impossible to describe without them. This new first chapter has been included at the request of students and at the suggestion of reviewers of the first edition. Structural formulae do not appear in subsequent chapters, all of which have in the most part been rewritten to include recent progress in these areas.

It is a pleasure to acknowledge the contributions from our colleagues (I.A.M., J.B. and D.J.H.) who were asked to write chapters on their specialist areas. All three teach in the medical course in Nottingham and have helped in its development. These chapters have broadened the scope of the text and hopefully improve its relevance to preclinical and junior clinical students. The inclusion of more clinical material should also be useful in this regard. It also reflects the changing interests of one of us (M.B.) in progressing from medical student to consultant physician since the first edition!

We are grateful to Deborah Briggs for preparing the manuscript from what at times were illegible originals and to Current Medical Literature for permission to adapt diagrams for Chapter 8.

David A. White
Michael Baxter
1993

Contents

List of Contributors

E Joan Bassey
Senior Lecturer in Exercise Physiology, Department of Physiology and Pharmacology, University of Nottingham, Medical School, Nottingham, UK

Michael Baxter
Consultant Endocrinologist, St Peter's Hospital, Chertsey, Surrey, UK

David J Hosking
Consultant Physician, City Hospital, Nottingham, UK

Ian A MacDonald
Professor of Metabolic Physiology, Department of Physiology and Pharmacology, University of Nottingham Medical School, Nottingham, UK

David White
Senior Lecturer, Department of Biochemistry, University of Nottingham Medical School, Nottingham, UK

1

Hormones: biosynthesis and mechanisms of action

Hormones may be defined as molecules which are synthesized by specific tissues and transported via the bloodstream to other specific target tissues where they elicit a response. The magnitude of this response is concentration related and the sensitivity of a tissue to a given hormone concentration is governed by the number of specific receptors on the tissue surface or, in the case of steroid hormones, in the cytosol. Hormones may be divided into four groups which reflect their structure and biosynthetic route:

1. Polypeptides, e.g. insulin, glucagon, growth factors.
2. Hormones derived from tyrosine, e.g. adrenaline, thyroxine.
3. Hormones derived from cholesterol, e.g. corticosteroids, sex hormones.
4. Products of arachidonic acid metabolism, e.g. prostaglandins, leuko-trienes.

Biosynthesis of hormones

Polypeptide hormones

Peptide hormones are translated from their messenger RNA (m-RNA) on the rough endoplasmic reticulum and translocation of the nascent polypeptide into the lumen of the endoplasmic reticulum is directed through the signal peptide encoded at the 3′ end of the m-RNA. This signal sequence is not normally found in the mature hormone, being cleaved from the primary translation product cotranslationally. Further post translational processing may occur during passage through the smooth endoplasmic reticulum, Golgi and secretory vesicles as illustrated in Fig. 1.1 for insulin and parathyroid hormone (parathormone; PTH). The mature hormone is released from the secretory granules during exocytosis arising from appropriate stimulation of the tissue. The m-RNA for PTH encodes a polypeptide of 115 amino acids, preproparathormone. Cotranslational cleavage of the signal sequence of 25 amino acids by the signal peptidase yields proparathormone which loses a further 6 amino acids by post-translational cleavage during packaging through the Golgi and the 84 amino acid parent hormone is stored in secretory vesicles. Interestingly

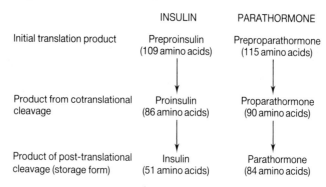

Fig. 1.1 Processing of nascent insulin and parathormone

only the first 34 amino acids are required for biological activity suggesting that further proteolysis might occur after release from the parathyroid gland. Similarly, insulin is synthesized as a single polypeptide chain, preproinsulin, and a signal sequence of 23 amino acids is cleaved cotranslationally to yield proinsulin. This undergoes post-translational cleavage, involving excision of the C-peptide, and disulphide bond formation, both intra- and inter-chain, to form the dimeric parent hormone.

In the absence of stimulated release of the stored peptide hormone it appears that much of it is degraded in the tissue in which it is synthesized.

Hormones synthesized from tyrosine

Catecholamines

Catecholamines are synthesized from tyrosine by chromaffin cells of the adrenal medulla and neurones of the central and peripheral nervous tissue (Fig. 1.2). The rate limiting step in this synthesis is the first one, hydroxylation of tyrosine by tyrosine hydroxylase to 3,4-dihydroxyphenylalanine (Dopa). This is feed-back inhibited by dopamine and noradrenaline. Decarboxylation of Dopa by the pyridoxal phosphate requiring enzyme Dopa decarboxylase then yields Dopamine, which undergoes further hydroxylation by a copper-dependent mixed-function oxidase, Dopamine β-hydroxylase, to noradrenaline. The final step, formation of adrenaline requires N-methylation of noradrenaline by phenylethanolamine S-methyltransferase using S-adenosylmethionine as donor of the methyl group. This enzyme is induced by glucocorticoids. The subcellular distribution of the enzyme activities is shown in Fig. 1.3. Formation of Dopa and Dopamine occurs in the cytoplasm prior to concentration of Dopamine into storage vesicles. Hydroxylation of Dopamine to noradrenaline takes place in the vesicle and conversion of noradrenaline to adrenaline requires release of the stored noradrenaline into the cytoplasm for N-methylation. Adrenaline is then transported into separate storage vesicles. In both storage vesicles the catecholamines are stored as Mg^{++}-ATP complexes with membrane proteins (chromagranins) and are released by exocytosis on stimulation. The action of catecholamines is terminated by uptake into the target cell followed by metabolism primarily to vanillyl mandelic acid.

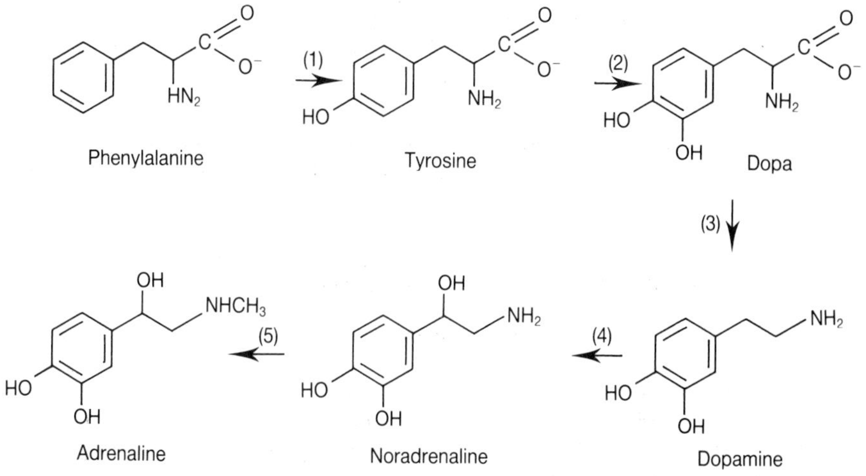

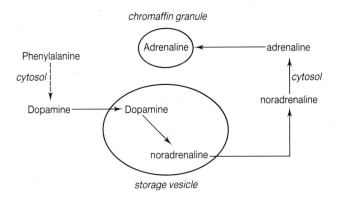

Fig. 1.2 Biosynthesis of Catecholamines
(1) Phenylalanine hydroxylase; (2) Tyrosine hydroxylase; (3) Dopa carboxylase; (4) Dopamine-β-hydroxylase; (5) Phenylethanolamine N-methyltransferase.

Thyroxine and triiodothyronine

Thyroxine is released from the thyroid gland on stimulation by thyroid stimulating hormone (TSH). Its precursor, thyroglobulin, is a high molecular weight glycoprotein (mol. wt. 660 kDa) containing 140 tyrosine residues of which 25 are iodinated during storage in the follicular lumen. Post translational modification of this protein involves the coupling of intra-chain iodotyrosines to leave a serine residue in the peptide linkage, and hydrolysis of the protein yields tetraiodothyronine (thyroxine, T_4) (Fig. 1.4). The active form of the thyroid

Fig. 1.3 Subcellular distribution of the enzymes of adrenaline biosynthesis

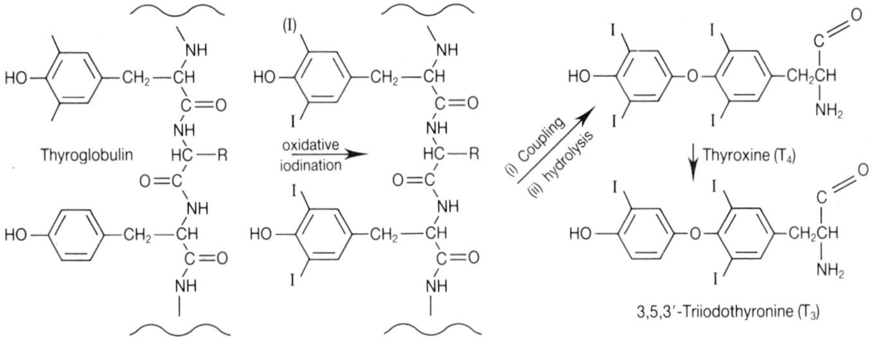

Fig. 1.4 Biosynthesis of thyroid hormones

hormone is triiodothyronine (T_3), formed from thyroxine by deiodination. Most of the T_3 and T_4 in the plasma is bound to an hepatically-synthesized glycoprotein, thyroxine-binding globulin (TBG); only the small unbound fraction is responsible for biological activity.

Steroid hormones

The major steroid-secreting tissues, adrenal cortex, gonads, placenta, synthesize steroid hormones from cholesterol stored in the tissue as cholesterol ester. Free cholesterol derived predominantly from hydrolysis of LDL-borne cholesterol ester or from *de novo* synthesis from acetyl coenzyme A, is esterified under the action of acylcoenzyme A: cholesterol acyltransferase (ACAT) (see Chapter 8). Steroid hormone synthesis requires activation of a cholesterylester hydrolase to release free cholesterol which is transported into the mitochodrion for further metabolism. The common intermediate in steroid biosynthesis from cholesterol is pregnenolone, formed in three steps catalysed by the mitochondrial enzyme desmolase and leads to the loss of a six-carbon fragment, isocaproic aldehyde, from the side chain of cholesterol. This process, which is stimulated by ACTH, involves hydroxylation of adjacent carbons (C_{20} and C_{22}) followed by oxidative cleavage between these carbons. The hydroxylations are catalysed by cytochrome P_{450}-dependent mixed-function oxidase activities. Conversion of pregnenolone to progesterone occurs extra-mitochodrially through oxidation of the original C_3 hydroxyl of cholesterol and isomerization of the Δ_5 double bond to Δ_4 (Fig. 1.5). This shuttling of the intermediates of steroid synthesis into and out of the mitochondrion continues as some of the hydroxylases which catalyse subsequent metabolic steps are cytosolic while others are mitochondrial. Cortisol is synthesized in the zona fasciculata of the adrenal cortex by hydroxylations at C_{17}, C_{21} and C_{11} of progesterone. Conversion of progesterone to aldosterone in the zona glomerulosa requires hydroxylations at C_{21}, C_{11} and

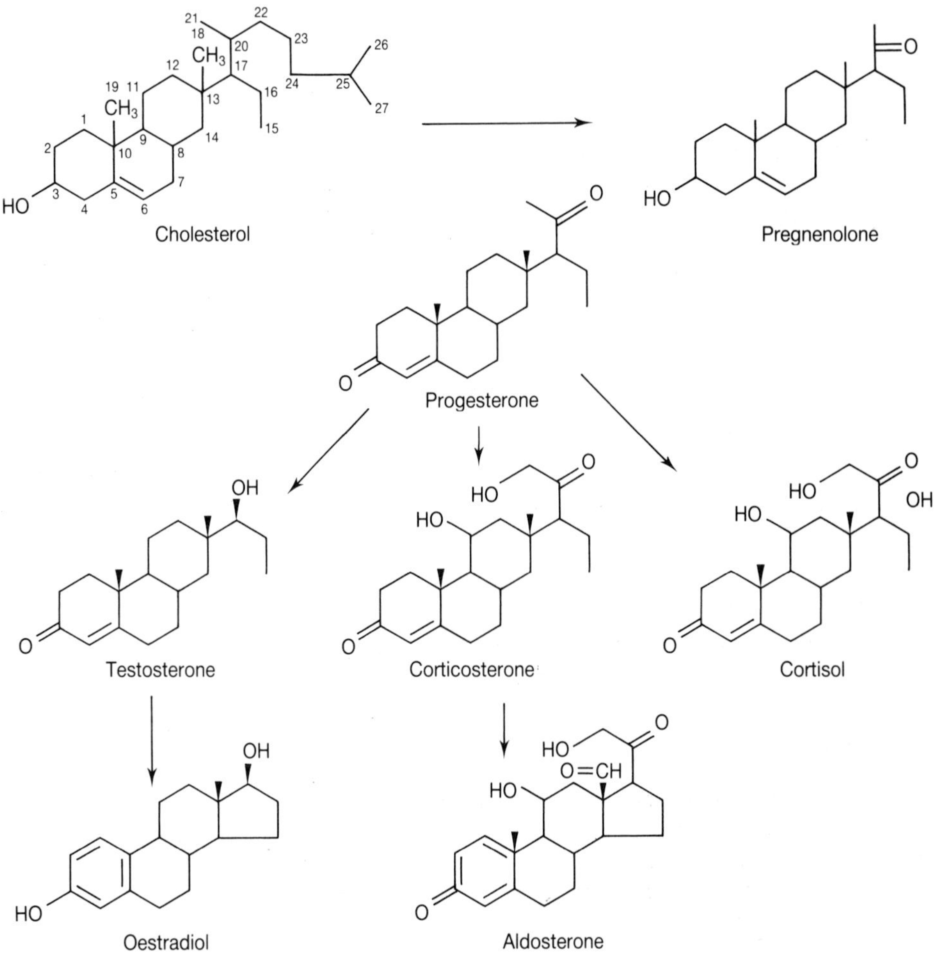

Fig. 1.5 Biosynthesis of steroid hormones from cholestrol

C_{18}, the latter two hydroxylations occurring in the mitochondrion. Although the synthesis of both the glucocorticoid (C_{21}) and mineralocorticoid (C_{21}) hormones occurs in the adrenal cortex their sub-tissue distribution allows for quite independent control systems; the renin-angiotensin system for aldosterone (see Chapter 10) and ACTH for cortisol.

Synthesis of the sex hormones may also take place in the adrenal cortex but occurs primarily in the gonads. The female sex hormones (C_{18}) are formed via the major male hormone testosterone (C_{19}). Again progesterone is a key intermediate which undergoes hydroxylation at C_{17} by a 17-hydroxylase followed by the loss of a two-carbon side chain at the same carbon to yield androstenedione. Further reduction at C_{17} yields testosterone. In the ovary and placenta, hydroxylation of testosterone at C_{19}, aromatization of the A ring and loss of carbon 10 yields 17β-oestradiol and similar reactions on androstenedione give rise to oestrone.

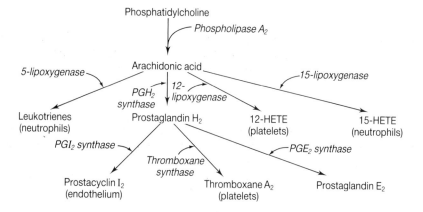

Fig. 1.6 Metabolism of phospholipid-derived arachidonic acid

The hydrophobic nature of steroid hormones requires that they be transported in the circulation bound to proteins; transcortin, a specific α-globulin synthesized in the liver, for cortisol, albumin for aldosterone and sex hormone-binding globulin (SHBG, a β-globulin) for sex hormones. Steroid hormones are inactivated by metabolism to products which render them more water soluble, allowing conjugation with sulphate or glucuronic acid and facilitating their excretion via the kidney.

Products of arachidonic metabolism

A number of biologically active peptides (e.g. cytokines) stimulate the release and metabolism of arachidonic acid derived from membrane phospholipids. This involves the initial action of a phospholipase A_2 on the intact phospholipid or possibly a lipase action on diacylglycerol produced by phospholipase C-catalysed hydrolysis of phosphatidylinositol bisphosphate (PIP_2: see later). The possible fates of arachidonic acid through four pathways in a variety of tissues are shown in Fig. 1.6.

Cyclooxygenase pathway

The classical prostaglandins are formed by the initial action of the prostaglandin endoperoxide synthase which exhibits cyclooxygenase and peroxidase activity. The cyclooxygenase catalyses the incorporation of two molecules of oxygen into the fatty acid and formation of a cyclopentane ring (PGG_2) while the peroxidase reduces PGG_2 to PGH_2. Non-steroidal antiinflammatory agents inhibit the cyclooxygenase, and aspirin (acetylsalicylic acid) causes irreversible inhibition by acetylating the enzyme. PGH_2 is the common precursor for prostaglandin E_2, prostacyclin I_2 and thromboxane A_2; the particular product formed is dependent on the enzyme complement of the individual tissue. Thus the principal metabolite of PGH_2 is prostacyclin I_2 in vascular endothelial cells and PGE_2 in for example the kidney, while thromboxane A_2 is a major product in the platelet.

(a) 12-Lipoxygenase.

Platelets also contain a 12-lipoxygenase which converts arachidonic acid to 12-hydroperoxy-eicosa-5,8,10,14-tetraenoic acid (12-HPETE). This can undergo further reduction to the 12-hydroxy derivative (12-HETE).

(b) 15-Lipoxygenase.

Neutrophils contain a 15-lipoxygenase which converts arachidonic acid to 15-hydroperoxy-eicosa-tetraenoic acid (15–HPETE) and this undergoes reduction to the 15-hydroxy derivative (15-HETE). This enzyme and its products may be important in the formation and development of atherosclerotic lesions (see Chapter 8).

(c) 5-Lipoxygenase.

The 5-lipoxygenase pathway found in neutrophils, eosinophils, monocytes, mast cells and keratinocytes gives rise to leukotrienes (LT) (the slow reacting substance (SRS-A) of anaphylaxis). The addition of glutathione by a specific glutathione transferase to leukotriene B_4 is important for many of the biological actions of leukotrienes, including contraction of respiratory, vascular and intestinal smooth muscles.

   All of the arachidonic acid derived products appear to bind to specific plasma membrane receptors and stimulate the formation of cAMP via activation of adenylate cyclase.

Mechanisms of action of hormones

Since hormones by definition are carried in the blood and have intracellular actions, signals which trigger intracellular responses must be transmitted across the plasma membrane of the target cell. Two quite different signalling pathways are apparent (Fig. 1.7). For instance, the interaction of peptide hormones, growth factors, neurotransmitters and arachidonic acid derivatives with plasma membrane receptors stimulates the synthesis of chemically distinct intracellular second messengers and subsequently the activation of protein kinases which elicit the metabolic response. Thus theoretically, the binding of a single hormone molecule/to its receptor could give rise to many intracellular second messenger molecules and this amplification of the original signal is an essential feature of this pathway. Steroid hormones and thyroid hormone on the other hand are lipid soluble and cross the plasma membrane before binding to intracellular receptors and exerting their regulatory actions in the nucleus.

Generation of second messengers

3′, 5′-Cyclic adenosine monophosphate (cAMP)

The adrenaline-sensitive β_2-adrenergic receptor and many peptide hormone

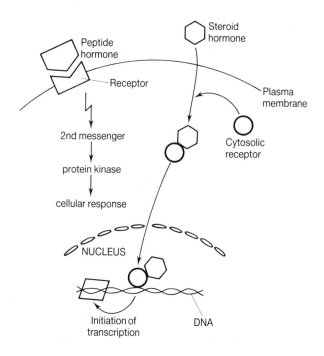

Fig. 1.7 Signalling pathways of peptide and steroid hormones

receptors such as the calcitonin receptor consist of a single polypeptide chain with seven membrane spanning domains. Binding of the ligand to the receptor causes activation or inhibition of adenylate cyclase via guanine nucleotide regulatory proteins (G-proteins) (Fig. 1.8) thereby changing the intracellular concentration of cAMP. These G-proteins are heterotrimers consisting of a guanine nucleotide binding α-chain (mol. wt. 39–52 kDa), a β-chain (35–36 kDa) and a small γ-chain (8 kDa). In the unstimulated state the G-protein binds GDP through interaction with the α-subunit. Binding of hormone to the extracellular site on the receptor induces a conformational change such that it interacts with the G_S protein causing dissociation of GDP and its replacement with GTP. The α-GTP complex then dissociates from the β- and γ-subunits and moves through the membrane to stimulate adenylate cyclase. The α-subunit also has intrinsic GTPase and hydrolysis of GTP terminates the activation of activity of adenylate cyclase and reformation of the trimeric G-protein. A similar chain of events occurs for the inhibitory receptor. The G_i protein associated with this system has identical β- and γ-subunits to the stimulatory G-protein. However, receptor activation and formation of the α-GTP complex inhibits adenylate cyclase. The importance of the GTP hydrolysis in terminating the response is shown by the actions of cholera toxin and pertussis toxin. Cholera toxin causes ADP-ribosylation of the α-subunit of the stimulatory G_S protein, preventing GTPase activity and thereby causing irreversible activation of adenylate cyclase. This action in the intestine results in the massive secretion of water and sodium ions and is responsible for the severe

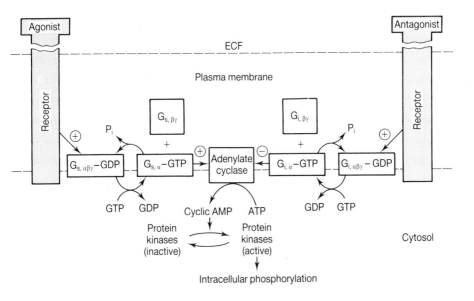

Fig. 1.8 Regulation of adenylate cyclase activity. See text for explanation. Abbreviations: ECF, extracellular fluid, ATP, adenosine 5'-triphosphate: P, orthophosphate

dehydration and salt depletion characteristic of cholera. Pertussis toxin also causes ADP-ribosylation but of the α-subunit of the inhibitory G_i protein, thus preventing the interaction of G_i with the receptor and the consequent inhibition of adenylate cyclase. Again adenylate cyclase acts in an unregulated manner. Interestingly, in cells where more than one hormone give rise to an increase in cAMP, the hormones appear to use a communal adenylate cyclase rather than have their own discrete enzyme and there may be competition for the limited amount of enzyme.

In eukaryotic cells probably all of the physiological effects of cAMP are mediated by cAMP-dependent protein kinases (PK-A), tetrameric proteins consisting of two catalytic and two regulatory subunits. When the intracellular cAMP concentration is raised cAMP binds to the regulatory subunits and induces a conformational change which causes dissociation of these subunits from the complex and allows the catalytic subunits to phosphorylate serine and threonine residues on target proteins (e.g. phosphorylase and glycogen synthetase). In some neuroendocrine cells the catalytic subunits of PK-A may translocate from the perinuclear–Golgi region into the nucleus and catalyse the phosphorylation, and thereby activation, of transcription regulatory factors. Thus, in this instance cAMP may stimulate gene transcription.

Metabolites of phosphatidylinositol-bisphosphate (PIP$_2$)

Phosphatidylinositol-bisphosphate is a minor component of the phospholipids of the plasma membrane which on hydrolysis through the action of

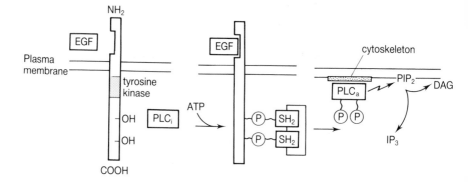

Fig. 1.9 Activation of PLC by EGF-mediated tyrosine kinase action. Binding of EGF causes autophosphorylation of the receptor which then forms a complex with PLC. PLC undergoes phosphorylation, conformational change and activation, allowing it to interact with the cytoskeleton and hydrolyse membrane bound PIP_2. PLC_i-inactive; PLC_a-active

phospholipase C (PLC) yields diacylglycerol and inositol (1,4,5)-trisphosphate, both of which may act as second messengers. There are at least four different species of mammalian PLC; PLC-γ_1 appears to be expressed in all mammalian tissues. Hormonal activation of PLC may be via a guanine nucleotide regulatory protein as for cAMP production, or via a receptor with intrinsic tyrosine kinase activity. These latter receptors (e.g. epidermal growth factor (EGF) receptor) contain a single membrane spanning domain and probably undergo oligomerization during signal transduction. Binding of ligand to the extracellular domain of the receptor stimulates the intracellular tyrosine kinase domain to catalyse autophosphorylation of the receptor allowing PLC-γ_1 to bind to it (Fig. 1.9). PLC-γ_1 contains specific domains SH2 and SH3 (which show sequence homology with domains of the *src* oncogene) that allow it to interact with first, the phosphorylated receptor (SH2) and second, the cytoskeleton (SH3). The receptor tyrosine kinase activity also catalyses the phosphorylation and activation of PLC-γ_1. This probably involves some conformational change which causes the enzyme to dissociate from the receptor and bind to the cytosolic surface of the plasma membrane through interaction of the SH3 domain with actin in the cytoskeleton. The activated PLC-γ_1 can then hydrolyse membrane-bound PIP_2 to inositol trisphosphate (IP_3) and diacylglycerol (DAG). PLC-γ_1 is thought to be deactivated by a tyrosine phosphatase.

Inositol trisphosphate

Inositol trisphosphate (IP_3) is water soluble and is responsible for the regulation of the concentration of intracellular calcium. IP_3 derived from PIP_2 by the action of PLC-γ_1 mediates the release of calcium from an intracellular storage compartment similar to the sarcoplasmic reticulum of muscle cells (Fig. 1.10). Calcium in this compartment appears to be bound to proteins (such as calsequestrin) which exhibit high capacity, low affinity binding sites.

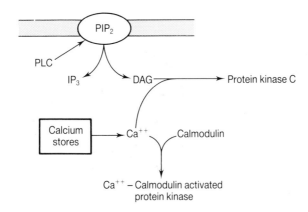

Fig. 1.10 Actions of the hydrolysis products of phosphatidylinositol bisphosphate (PIP$_2$) (PLC phospholipase C: DAG, diacylglycerol: IP$_3$, inositol trisphosphate)

Release of this stored calcium into the cytosol raises the intracellular calcium concentration from its homoeostatic submicromolar range to the micromolar range and activates calcium dependent processes.

Another possible source of calcium is extracellular fluid. The calcium concentration gradient across the plasma membrane is in the same direction as sodium but is at least four orders of magnitude greater and this gradient is maintained by the action of membrane-bound calcium pumps. It has been suggested that calcium gates in the plasma membrane might be opened by inositol polyphosphates derived from PIP$_2$ hydrolysis and phosphorylation of the released IP$_3$. This too would lead to an increase in cytosolic calcium. Mitochondria also have a large capacity for calcium storage but the contribution of this organelle to the regulation of cytosolic calcium concentration is not known.

For many calcium-activated processes, however, it is not calcium *per se* but a calcium–protein complex which is responsible for the activation. A number of calcium-binding proteins have been reported but perhaps calmodulin is the best described. This small globular protein (mol. wt. 16.7 kDa) has four calcium binding sites and calcium binding causes a conformational change increasing its α-helical content. As the intracellular calcium concentration rises above the dissociation constant for the calcium–calmodulin complex the complex, which has no intrinsic enzyme activity, binds to and activates enzymes and membrane transport systems including the calcium pump (Fig. 1.11). In this way the calcium–calmodulin complex initiates calcium removal from the cytosol and limits the duration of the calcium signal. A particular example of the action of the calcium–calmodulin complex is its role in the promotion of glycogenolysis in skeletal muscle (Fig. 1.12). Contraction of the muscle requires ATP generated by glycogenolysis and subsequent glycolysis. Stimulation of the muscle causes release of calcium from the sarcoplasmic reticulum, raising the cytosolic concentration of the cation. Calcium binds to troponin C, activating the actomyosin ATPase and initiating muscle contraction. Calcium also binds to both free calmodulin but particularly to that which is the δ-subunit of phosphorylase

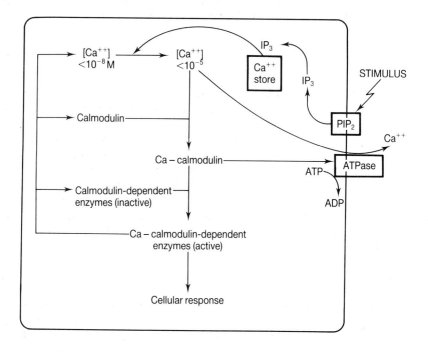

Fig. 1.11 The involvement of calmodulin in stimulus-response coupling

kinase. Calcium binding by the δ-subunit activates the kinase and promotes the phosphorylation of glycogen phosphorylase and glycogen synthetase (see Chapter 2). It is likely that a second molecule of calmodulin or troponin C is required *in vivo* to bind the phosphorylase–synthetase complex to the myofibril giving an on-tap feed of ATP from glycolysis, for contraction. Again, the action

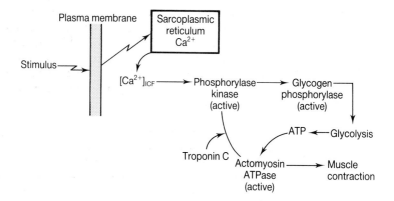

Fig. 1.12 Involvement of the calcium-calmodulin complex in glycogen metabolism and muscle contraction

of the calcium-calmodulin-activated calcium pump will reduce the intracellular calcium concentration and return the system to homoeostasis.

Diacylglycerol

The other product of phospholipase C-catalysed hydrolysis of PIP_2 is diacylglycerol. This can serve as a provider of arachidonic acid for eicosanoid synthesis shown above, or in the intact form as an activator of a specific calcium-dependent protein kinase, protein kinase-C (PK-C or C-kinase). Activation of the plasma /membrane-bound PK-C involves proteolysis yielding a soluble Ca^{2+}/lipid-dependent enzyme that is able to phosphorylate cellular proteins, including transcriptional regulators and lead to altered rates of transcription of a number of genes. It is not known whether the soluble PK-C translocates to the nucleus before phosphorylation of the transcriptional regulators or that translocation of the regulator occurs after its cytosolic phosphorylation by PK-C.

Steroid hormones

The response to steroid hormones and thyroid hormones involves actions on transcription of DNA in the cell nucleus and is mediated by protein receptors. Binding of the hormone to the cytosolic receptor causes dimerization of the receptor and /promotes translocation of the hormone–dimer complex from the cytosol to the nucleus where it binds to regulatory elements upstream of the particular gene to be regulated. Structural studies have defined three features common to a number of steroid receptors, a variable N-terminus, a short, well-conserved central domain and a complex C-terminus (Fig. 1.13). The ligand binding site and dimerization sites are both located in the C-terminal domain, as is the sequence which signals the movement of the receptor into the nucleus. The central domain contains a helix-turn-helix motif and a cysteine-rich sequence allowing the formation of two 'zinc fingers', features common to many DNA-binding proteins. The zinc finger motifs appear /to be responsible for maintaining the structure of the DNA-binding domain and allowing the correct presentation of the DNA-recognition helices which bind in adjacent major grooves on one face of the DNA-double helix (Fig. 1.14). While variations in the amino acid sequence of the central domain give rise to discrimination in binding sites on DNA, other amino acids are highly conserved and mutation

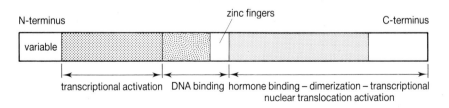

Fig. 1.13 Proposed general structural features of steroid and thyroid hormone receptors

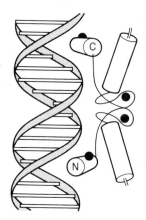

Fig. 1.14 Schematic model of the protein-DNA complex formed between the DNA-binding domain of two receptor molecules and their palindromic recognition sequence. Solid circles represent zinc atoms; N = N-terminus: C-carboxyregion of DNA-recognition helices. (Reproduced with permission Schwabe, JWR and Rhodes D, TIBS 16 (1991) 291-296 copyright 1991 Elsevier Science Publishers UK)

may lead to a receptor with greatly reduced DNA binding affinity. Such a mutation is/responsible for vitamin D-resistant hypocalcaemic rickets, where $1,25(OH)_2D$ can bind to its receptor but this complex cannot switch on the synthesis of the calcium transport proteins required for intestinal uptake of dietary calcium (see Chapter 9).

The sequence of events which gives rise to activation of transcription is shown in Fig. 1.15. Plasma-borne hormone is recognized by some receptor on the target cell and moves into the cytosol. The cytosolic ligand-free receptor protein

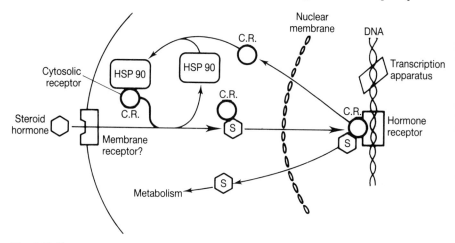

Fig. 1.15 Transport of steroid hormones to the nucleus
S = steroid hormone; C.R. = cytosolic receptor

which exists as a monomer undergoes some allosteric structural change on ligand binding such that it dimerizes and translocates to the nucleus. The dimer binds to short palindromic sequences (hormone response elements) which flank the hormone responsive genes and activate transcription of the particular gene. Such a scheme requires of course that there are steroid-free receptors in the cytoplasm to accept the hormone. It has been suggested that the unoccupied receptor forms a macromolecular complex with one of the heat shock proteins (HSP 90) in the cytoplasm such that translocation of the receptor into the nucleus cannot occur until it is released from the complex by the binding of the hormone. In this way the process is akin to the cAMP-mediated pathway which leads to activation of the protein kinase only after the binding of cAMP to the regulatory subunits.

2

Nutrition and energy metabolism

Nutrition

Whilst it is beyond the scope of this book to present a detailed account of nutritional aspects of metabolism, a brief description is worthwhile. Most readers will be aware of the need to consume a 'balanced diet', and that this comprises adequate amounts of fat, carbohydrate and protein (the macronutrients), vitamins and minerals (the micronutrients), water and fibre. Obviously, the macronutrients in the diet are the source of energy, and so are of particular importance in the consideration of normal and abnormal energy metabolism. However, many of the micronutrients are also important for normal energy metabolism, either as co-factors for enzyme activity (e.g. minerals such as Ca^{++}, Mg^{++} for ATPase) or as precursors of important intermediates (e.g. B vitamins such as riboflavin (flavin mononucleotides), nicotinic acid (NAD) and pantothenic acid (coenzyme A)).

Nutrient requirements

In order to maintain an adequate nutritional status it is vital that the consumption of nutrients balances their utilization. The existence of body stores of energy, vitamins and minerals means that a temporary inadequacy of the dietary intake of a nutrient does not immediately produce deficiency leading to disordered metabolism. Conversely, excess consumption of nutrients can lead to an increase in the size of the body store of that substance. We will concentrate in this book, on the energy requirements of an individual and the consequence of failing to match energy intake to those requirements, i.e. starvation and obesity.

Energy intake

Dietary energy is mainly derived from the fat, protein and carbohydrate contents of foodstuffs, although the average British adult obtains approximately 10 per cent of total energy intake from alcohol. The energy content (energy density) of these nutrients are given in Table 2.1, but it is worth remembering that very few foods/beverages contain these nutrients in their pure form – the water and fibre contents mean that the energy density of food can be substantially less than

Table 2.1   Energy content of main nutrients

	Energy content	
Nutrient	kJ/g	kcal/g
Fat	37	9
Carbohydrate	16	3.75
Protein	17	4
Ethanol	29	7

that of the primary nutrients (Table 2.2).

An individual's energy requirements are determined by body size, physical activity and stage of growth, and may be altered in situations such as pregnancy, infection and trauma. The regulation of energy intake, and its balancing to energy expenditure is considered in Chapter 3, after the biochemical aspects of energy metabolism have been outlined in this chapter.

Apart from rare metabolic defects which prevent the normal utilization of one of the major nutrients, an individual's energy requirements can, in theory, be met with any combination of protein, fat and carbohydrate. However, the utilization of protein as a fuel for energy metabolism is very inefficient, as the process of deamination of amino acids, urea production and excretion requires the expenditure of a substantial amount of energy and may place an excessive burden on renal function. In practice, the majority of dietary energy intake is obtained from fat and carbohydrate. In the diet of the average adult in the UK in 1990, fat provided between 40 and 45 per cent of 'non-alcohol' energy intake. This is somewhat higher than the recommendations made by numerous expert committees, where the consensus is that in order to reduce the incidence of obesity and atherosclerosis in the population, fat intakes should be below 35

Table 2.2   Energy and protein content of common foods

Food	Energy kcal/100g	Protein g/100g	Average portion	Energy kcal	Protein g
White bread	235	8.4	Slice (30g)	71	2.5
Brown bread	215	9.2	Slice (35g)	75	3.2
Hard cheese	412	25.5	10g	41	2.6
Full fat milk	66	3.2	Pint	378	18.4
Skimmed milk	33	3.3	Pint	189	18.9
Butter	737	0.5	10g	7	0.05
Red meat	613	11.9	Slice (45g)	142	5.4
White meat	148	24.8	1 breast	192	32.2
Fish	94	20.9	Fillet	113	25.1
Vegetables	42	3.3	90g	38	3.0
Baked beans	84	5.2	Small tin	189	11.7
Beer (bitter)	32	0.3	Pint	184	1.7

Table 2.3 Average estimated energy/protein requirements based on average weight adults

	Estimated protein intake (g/d)	Physical activity level	Estimated energy requirements MJ/d(kcal/d)
Women	45.0	Active	8.8 (2090)
		Sedentary	7.8 (1850)
Men	55.5	Active	11.4 (2710)
		Sedentary	10.1 (2400)

per cent of 'non-alcohol' energy intake (Table 2.3). Furthermore, the ideal diet for preventing the development of obesity and atherosclerosis would have most of the carbohydrates in the complex, starchy form (which also means that fibre intake would be high) and more than half of its fat in the polyunsaturated form (vegetables and fish oils) with a low saturated fat (animal fats) content.

Energy metabolism and its control

Homoeostasis may be defined as a state of physiological equilibrium produced by a balance of functions and of chemical composition within an organism. Two opposing metabolic processes contribute to such a state. Anabolism is the building process responsible for the biosynthesis of cellular macromolecules and energy storage whilst catabolism is the destructive metabolic process whereby complex molecules are broken into smaller molecules with a release of energy. Although both processes can be controlled independently, homoeostasis implies a balance between the two and this is maintained through the actions of hormones which coordinate and control tissue responses. Such control avoids the wasteful degradation of newly-synthesized macromolecules. Tissue responses may be acute, lasting of the order of a few minutes or chronic, of the order of hours or even days. Acute control involves the modification of enzyme activity by allosteric modulators or by covalent modification such as phosphorylation, whereas chronic control results in a change in enzyme amount arising from a change in enzyme synthesis and/or degradation (Fig. 2.1). A tissue may thus adapt its metabolism chronically after initial changes imposed as a result of acute effects.

Catabolism

The catabolic state, characterized by the degradation of stored fuel molecules, glycogen, triacylglycerol and protein, is one in which the plasma concentration of insulin is decreased while that of adrenaline, glucagon, glucocorticoids and growth hormone is increased (Table 2.4). Indeed this latter group of hormones exerts general catabolic effects and only insulin may be regarded as anabolic. Even growth hormone, whose name suggests anabolism, is anabolic only in the presence of raised insulin levels. It becomes catabolic when insulin levels

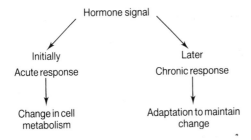

Fig. 2.1 Tissue response to hormone signals

are decreased or cortisol levels are increased.

The overall metabolic state of the body at a particular time depends on the ratio of anabolic to catabolic hormones with the response of a particular tissue dependent upon the concentration of the individual hormone and the relative number of its receptors in that tissue.

Fat catabolism

Fat is stored as triacylglycerol, predominantly in white adipose tissue from which free fatty acids are mobilized in times of metabolic need. Oxidation of the fatty acids, producing reducing equivalents for the generation of ATP, then takes place in other tissues to which the free fatty acids are transported.

Mobilization.

The release of free fatty acids from triacylglycerols (TAG) stored in adipose tissue is catalysed by a hormone-sensitive lipase which is subject to acute regulation by phosphorylation via the cAMP cascade described in Chapter 1. Binding of glucagon or adrenaline to their specific membrane receptors stimulates the synthesis of cAMP and activation of a protein kinase which in turn catalyses phosphorylation and activation of the lipase. More chronic regulation of the lipase activity is brought about by the synergistic actions of growth hormone and cortisol which increase enzyme amount (Fig. 2.2).

White adipose tissue has few mitochondria and consequently only a limited capacity for β-oxidation of free fatty acids. The excess free fatty acids thus leave the tissue and are transported as a fatty acid–albumin complex to other tissues such as heart, skeletal muscle, liver and kidney. Uptake and subsequent metabolism of the free fatty acids by these tissues is controlled by the blood concentration of the fatty acids. Two possible routes of metabolism may be followed, oxidation or resynthesis of triacylglycerol for VLDL assembly and the relative flow into each is dependent upon the hormonal state (Fig. 2.3). Thus, in most catabolic states, the bulk of the fatty acids are oxidized but in situations where there is a peripheral resistance to insulin, e.g. diabetes or trauma, hepatic synthesis of triacylglycerol may be significant. Little, if any, triacylglycerol resynthesis occurs in tissues other

Table 2.4 Hormonal changes in metabolic states

Hormonal changes	Metabolic effects	Hormonal changes	Metabolic effects
Insulin ↑ *(— means lots of sugar in blood)* Glucagon ↓ Adrenaline ↓ Cortisol ↓ (Glucocorticoids) Growth hormone ↑*	Increased formation of protein, glycogen and triacylglycerol Increased synthesis of fatty acids and sterols	Insulin ↓ Glucagon ↑ Adrenaline ↑ Cortisol ↑ (Glucocorticoids) Growth hormone ↑*	Increased mobilization and breakdown of glucose, fatty acids and amino acids liberated from tissue stores (glycogen, triacylglycerol and protein)

* Elevation of growth hormone in the presence of raised insulin concentrations is anabolic in effect, but is catabolic when insulin levels are decreased and cortisol levels raised.

Insulin lowers blood sugar

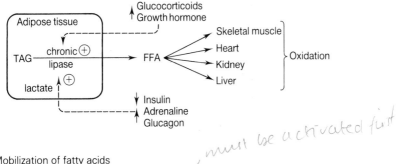

must be activated first

Fig. 2.2 Mobilization of fatty acids

than liver however, and the fatty acids undergo primarily β-oxidation in the mitochondria. Transport of the activated fatty acid into the mitochondrial inner membrane requires the formation of acylcarnitine (Fig. 2.4) on the mitochondrial inner membrane. This represents the slowest step in the overall oxidation process and is inhibited by malonylcoenzyme A, an intermediate in fatty acid synthesis (see p. 22). Thus, under anabolic conditions, where the malonyl-CoA concentration is raised, β-oxidation is inhibited. Under catabolic conditions however, where fatty acid synthesis is inhibited, the rate of β-oxidation is determined by the supply of fatty acids and the mitochondrial carnitine content. In a tissue such as muscle, where little fatty acid synthesis occurs, the rate of β-oxidation is dependent on the supply of fatty acids to the tissue which in turn reflects the rate of triacylglycerol breakdown in adipose tissue. The products of β-oxidation are acetylcoenzyme A and NADH.

Ketone body metabolism

Ketone bodies : produced when AcCoA is formed from βox" quicker than its consumption via TCAC

In man, increased lipolysis is accompanied by ketonaemia as the liver synthesizes ketone bodies (acetoacetate and 3-hydroxybutyrate) when β-oxidation proceeds at a rate which exceeds that at which acetyl-CoA enters the citric acid cycle. This process occurs only in the liver since it is the only tissue with the enzymes required for ketogenesis and has a limited citric acid cycle capacity. The stoichiometry of acetoacetate synthesis and the kinetic properties of the enzymes of the ketogenic pathway are such that the rate of acetoacetate synthesis is proportional to the square of the rate of β-oxidation. The rapid rate of β-oxidation produces an increase in the NADH/NAD+ ratio

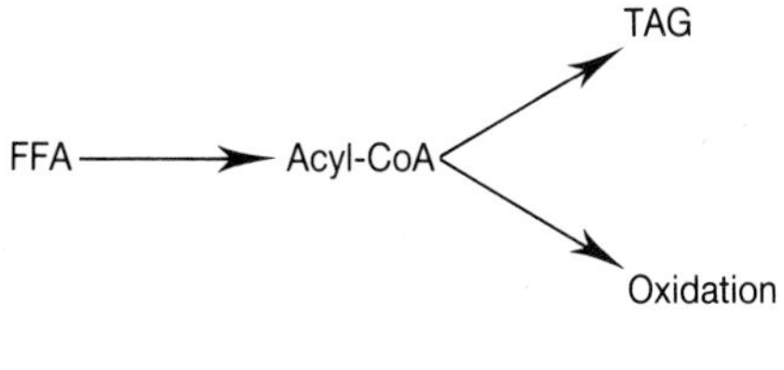

KB b/c liver: limited TCAC + ketogenic enzymes

TAG

FFA ⟶ Acyl-CoA ⟨

Oxidation

Fig. 2.3 Liver response to plasma FFA

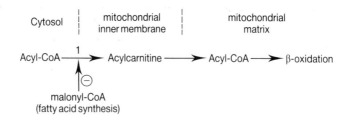

Fig. 2.4 Control of β-oxidation

which in turn slows down the citric acid cycle. In an attempt to regenerate NAD⁺ in the mitochondrion a significant proportion of acetoacetate (3-keto-butyrate) is reduced to 3-hydroxybutyrate with concomitant oxidation of NADH to NAD⁺.

Ketone bodies are used rapidly in extrahepatic tissues such as heart, skeletal muscle and kidney (Fig. 2.5), being converted first to acetoacetyl-CoA by a 3-ketoacyl-CoA transferase which catalyses the transfer of coenzymeA from succinyl-CoA (an intermediate of the citric acid cycle) to acetoacetate. The acetoacetyl-CoA is then hydrolysed to acetyl-CoA which is oxidized without limitation in these tissues. The liver itself cannot use ketone bodies as it lacks the 3-ketoacyl-CoA transferase. In brain, ketone bodies may become significant fuels when their plasma concentration rises sufficiently to allow rapid uptake by this tissue, e.g. during starvation. Thus ketone body production by the liver and their oxidation by extrahepatic tissues is increased by catabolic hormones which give rise to increased adipose tissue lipolysis and hepatic β-oxidation.

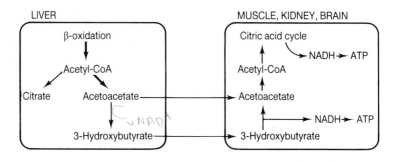

Fig. 2.5 Ketone body mobilization

Carbohydrate catabolism

Like fat catabolism, the catabolism of carbohydrate involves a two-stage process, the initial release of glucose units (glycogenolysis) from body stores followed by metabolism of these released glucose units (glycolysis).

Table 2.5   Consequences of glycogenolysis in liver and muscle

Hormone change		Tissue	Glycogen to glucose	Glycogen to pyruvate
Insulin	↓			
Adrenaline	↑	Liver	+ + +	− (by glucagon)
Glucagon	↑			
Insulin	↓	Muscle	Not occur	+ + +
Adrenaline	↑			

Glycogenolysis

Carbohydrate is stored primarily as glycogen, a polymer of glucose, in liver and muscle. Release of glucose units, as glucose-1-phosphate is controlled by the action of glycogen phosphorylase. Raised adrenaline or decreased insulin concentrations (i.e. increased catabolic to anabolic hormone ratio) cause a rapid mobilization of glucose units in liver and muscle whilst raised glucagon levels stimulate glycogenolysis in liver only (Table 2.5). The precise molecular mechanism of insulin action is still unclear but the consequences of a raised plasma adrenaline concentration on the activity of glycogen phosphorylase in muscle have been described in detail and a similar mechanism obtains for the action of glucagon in liver. A small rise in the plasma concentration of these hormones increases their binding to their specific receptors on target tissues and activates the synthesis of cAMP (see Chapter 1). The raised intracellular concentration of cAMP in turn initiates an enzyme cascade involving specific kinases and phosphatases which results in the net phosphorylation of the less active phosphorylase **b** to the more active phosphorylase **a** (Fig. 2.6). The effects of adrenaline in the liver however are not mediated via cAMP but via an increase in the intracellular free calcium concentration which causes a direct activation of phosphorylase **b** kinase (Chapter 1). A similar activation by raised cytosolic free calcium of phosphorylase **b** kinase can also occur in muscle as a result of a neural stimulus and cause glycogen breakdown independent of adrenaline stimulation.

The simultaneous phosphorylation of glycogen synthase causes its inactivation and minimizes the futile cycling of glucose units. Phosphorylase is also an allosteric enzyme and subject to further control by physiological effectors (Table 2.6). The active conformation of the enzyme is stabilized by phosphorylation even in the absence of an allosteric activator and only glucose is a significant inhibitor of the phosphorylated form.

Glycolysis

The glycolytic pathway where glucose (6 carbons) is broken down to pyruvate (3 carbons) is present in all tissues and can be used both catabolically for energy production (exercising muscle, red blood cell) or anabolically for lipid

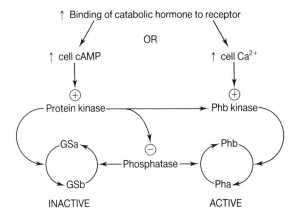

Fig. 2.6 Activation of phosphorylase (Ph) and inhibition of glycogen synthase (GS)

synthesis from glucose units (liver and adipose tissue). Under catabolic conditions glycolysis is active in those tissues which derive a significant proportion of their energy requirement from glucose (brain, muscle, red blood cells, but not liver). The source of glucose for glycolysis in this case is either endogenous glycogen or blood glucose which is derived from hepatic glycogen. The entry of glucose into adipose tissue and resting muscle requires insulin which recruits intracellular glucose transport molecules to the plasma membrane (Table 2.7). In working muscle however, glucose entry into the cell is less dependent on insulin such that glycolysis can proceed from exogenous glucose in exercise even under catabolic conditions (i.e. reduced insulin concentration).

In muscle, brain and red blood cells the rate of glycolysis is controlled at the level of phosphofructokinase (PFK) by allosteric effectors which reflect the energy charge (ATP/AMP ratio) of the tissue (Fig. 2.7). A sufficient supply of energy raises the ATP concentration relative to that of AMP and inhibits PFK. A raised ATP concentration also slows the citric acid cycle (p. 29) causing an increase in the concentration of cytosolic citrate. Citrate is another allosteric inhibitor of PFK and inhibition of this enzyme leads to an increase in glucose-6-phosphate which inhibits hexokinase, thereby decreasing the rate of entry of glucose into the pathway.

Table 2.6   Physiological effectors of phosphorylase

Phosphorylase form and activity		Inhibitor	Activator	Tissue where effect is important
b	Inactive without AMP	ATP Glucose-6-P	AMP	Muscle
b	Active without AMP	Glucose	–	Liver

Table 2.7 Effect of insulin on glucose transport across plasma membranes

Tissue	Stimulation by insulin
Liver	None
Brain	None
Muscle	+ + + but less in heavy exercise
Adipose	+ + +

In the catabolic state, the liver serves as a net supplier of glucose to the blood and besides stimulating glycogenolysis, glucagon also causes inhibition of glycolysis, thereby decreasing hepatic use of glucose. The glucagon-stimulated elevation of cAMP activates protein kinases which are responsible for the inhibition of glycolysis by first, phosphorylating pyruvate kinase such that it is inhibited by the prevailing phosphoenolpyruvate concentration and second, decreasing the intracellular concentration of fructose-2,6-bisphosphate (F-2,6P$_2$). Phosphofructokinase is a major regulatory enzyme of the glycolytic pathway and F-2,6P$_2$ is the most potent activator of this enzyme, antagonizing the allosteric inhibition of ATP and citrate. The decreased F-2,6P$_2$ concentration caused by the action of glucagon thus results in a decreased activity of PFK. Hepatic glycolysis is therefore inhibited at two sites (pyruvate kinase and PFK) by an elevated plasma glucagon (Fig. 2.8).

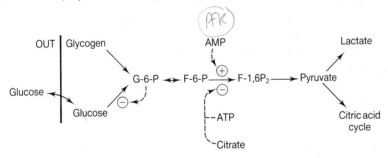

Fig. 2.7 Glycolysis in extrahepatic tissues

Pyruvate oxidation

The oxidation of pyruvate to acetyl-CoA is an irreversible process and because animal cells cannot synthesize glucose from two-carbon units (acetate) it represents a net loss of the body's carbohydrate reserves. Conservation of three-carbon units is essential when an exogenous supply of glucose is limited and thus pyruvate oxidation is closely regulated. The enzyme responsible for pyruvate oxidation is pyruvate dehydrogenase (PDH) which undergoes a cAMP independent phosphorylation–dephosphorylation cycle catalysed by a kinase and phosphatase respectively (Fig. 2.9). Insulin and a raised intracellular calcium concentration stimulate the phosphatase, thereby increasing the

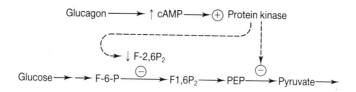

Fig. 2.8 Control of hepatic glycolysis

amount of active dephosphorylated PDH enzyme. The kinase on the other hand, is activated by raised acetyl-CoA and NADH concentrations, conditions which lead to inhibition of pyruvate oxidation. Thus pyruvate oxidation is inhibited by the decreased insulin concentrations of the catabolic state and also by an increased supply of acetyl-CoA from β-oxidation or when the redox state of the cell rises.

Gluconeogenesis Making Glucose.

Gluconeogenesis occurs only in liver and kidney. As the name implies, it is a synthetic process and therefore anabolic. However, it occurs only when the body is in an overall catabolic state, being part of the process by which glucose is generated from products of the breakdown of protein. Indeed, gluconeogenesis is stimulated by raised glucagon and glucocorticoid and decreased by raised insulin. The acute stimulation by glucagon and glucocorticoid is due to the removal of $F-2,6P_2$, the allosteric activator of PFK and inhibitor of fructose-1,6-bisphosphatase (FBPase) thereby activating gluconeogenesis and inhibiting glycolysis. As mentioned earlier, the lowered insulin concentration promotes the phosphorylation and consequent inhibition of pyruvate dehydrogenase which conserves three-carbon pyruvate (derived from lactate and alanine) for gluconeogenesis. Glycerol, derived from lipolysis in adipose tissue, is also an important three-carbon molecule for gluconeogenesis, entering the pathway after phosphorylation to glycerol-3-phosphate and oxidation to dihydroxyacetone phosphate. Chronic changes in a prolonged catabolic state lead to increased amounts of the 'key' enzymes (1,2,3 in Fig. 2.10) of gluconeogenesis. The whole process is limited by substrate supply and

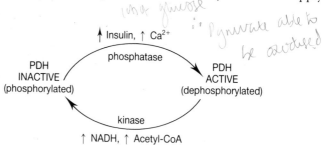

Fig. 2.9 Control of pyruvate dehydrogenase

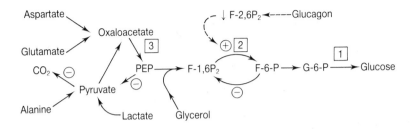

Fig. 2.10 Gluconeogenesis. 1. Glucose-6-phosphatase; 2. Fructose 1:6 bisphosphatase; 3. Phosphoenolpyruvate carboxykinase

can be inhibited by high redox states ($NADH/NAD^+$ ratios) such as occurs in excess alcohol ingestion where the oxidation of ethanol to ethanal and finally ethanoate (acetate) by alcohol dehydrogenase requires the concomitant reduction of NAD^+ to NADH. The brandy brought to the cold and hungry lost skier may be welcome psychologically but sandwiches and a few sugar lumps would be better metabolically!

Protein and amino acid catabolism

An average adult in nitrogen balance degrades about 300–400 g of protein each day and this is replaced by newly synthesized protein. Even in excessive catabolic states (e.g. major burns and infection, Chapter 5) the amino acids derived from protein degradation never provide more than about 20 per cent of the metabolic fuel requirements. Again, raised concentrations of the catabolic hormones, glucocorticoids and glucagon stimulate breakdown of protein, the former in muscle and liver whilst the latter only in liver. The precise mechanism of these actions is unknown but raised insulin is antagonistic, i.e. inhibits protein degradation and the net rate of protein degradation to amino acids represents a balance between the anabolic and catabolic hormones (Fig 2.11).

Amino acid catabolism

1) removal of a gp
2) catabolism of c skeleton

The initial reaction in the breakdown of amino acids involves the removal of the unwanted α-amino group by pyridoxal phosphate-dependent transamination to a ketoacid and catabolism of the remaining carbon skeleton. The α-amino group NH_3 is eventually converted to urea and excreted (Fig. 2.12). These processes are regulated acutely by the concentration of substrate and therefore ultimately by the net rate of protein breakdown which supplies the amino acid substrates. Both glucagon and glucocorticoids increase amino acid catabolism chronically by increasing the amounts of the enzymes involved in catabolism. Glucagon

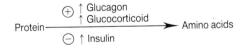

Fig. 2.11 Protein degradation

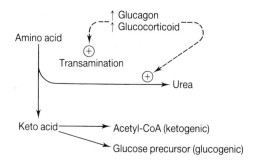

Fig. 2.12 Amino acid catabolism

also stimulates the uptake and subsequent metabolism of circulating alanine by the liver. This is of major importance in the catabolism of protein-derived amino acids. The liver is the only tissue capable of synthesizing urea from the α-amino groups derived from amino acids in the muscle, and alanine serves as a transporter of the three-carbons required for gluconeogenesis and of waste nitrogen for excretion as urea. This gives rise to the glucose–alanine cycle (Fig. 2.13). The control of the breakdown of the carbon skeleton of amino acids depends on the nature of the α-ketoacid produced on transamination. Most are converted to citric acid cycle or glycolytic (and therefore gluconeogenetic) intermediates and are known as glucogenic amino acids. The branched chain amino acids, after transamination, undergo decarboxylation by an enzyme complex similar to pyruvate dehydrogenase which is also under control by a kinase and phosphatase. Under catabolic conditions leucine is metabolized solely to ketone bodies and is the only purely ketogenic amino acid.

Control of the citric acid cycle and oxidative phosphorylation

Oxidation of acetate in the citric acid cycle generates reducing equivalents in the form of NADH and $FADH_2$ at the four dehydrogenase reactions. Since the amount of NAD^+ in the mitochondrion is limited, the rate at which the cycle operates is governed by the concentration of NAD^+ which in turn is dependent on the reoxidation of NADH via the electron transport chain. Thus the $NADH/NAD^+$ ratio exerts important control over the cycle (Fig. 2.14). Further, a high rate of acetyl-CoA input, from glycolysis and β-oxidation, into the cycle produces a raised citrate level in the mitochondrion. Excess citrate flows out of the mitochondrion into the cytosol, inhibiting glycolysis at the level of PFK and slowing the citric acid cycle by reducing substrate supply. Thus in times of increased fat breakdown, with β-oxidation supplying acetyl-CoA, carbohydrate utilization is spared at the expense of fat. In the liver, the maximal activity of citrate synthase is low such that when β-oxidation occurs at a high rate, excess acetyl-CoA is directed to ketone body production.

Electron transport in mitochondria is normally tightly coupled to the synthesis of ATP. The series of redox reactions in the electron transport chain generates energy which is used to pump protons out of the mitochondrial matrix

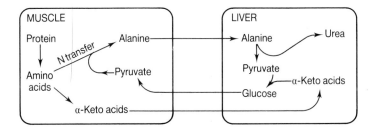

Fig. 2.13 Glucose alanine cycle

and sets up a proton gradient across the mitochondrial inner membrane which is dissipated by proton re-entry into the matrix via the ATP synthase complex and synthesis of ATP. In this coupled state the rate of electron transport is determined by the rate of phosphorylation which in turn is dependent on the matrix concentration of ADP. With a limited total adenine nucleotide content in the matrix the rate of electron transport and thus the $NADH/NAD^+$ ratio is governed by the ADP/ATP ratio. At any one time therefore, the cellular requirement for ATP determines the concentration of mitochondrial NADH and ultimately controls the dehydrogenases of the citric acid cycle. Uncoupling of phosphorylation from electron transport allows electron transport and consequently the citric acid cycle to proceed at a faster rate. In this case the energy generated in the redox reactions of the electron transport chain is dissipated as heat, a process which can occur in brown adipose tissue (Chapter 3).

Anabolism

The anabolic state is characterized by a rise in the concentration of insulin relative to that of the catabolic hormones, glucagon, catecholamines and glucocorticoids. For example, immediately after a meal, particularly one enriched in carbohydrates, diet-derived glucose and amino acids and also gastrointestinal (GI) peptides stimulate the release of insulin from the β-cells of the

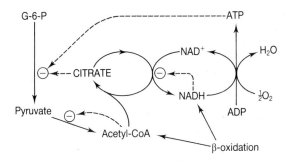

Fig. 2.14 Limitation of citric acid cycle rate by ATP via NADH

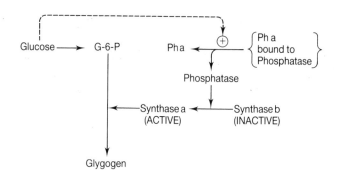

Fig. 2.15 Glucose stimulation of glycogen synthesis in liver

pancreas. Insulin then promotes the synthesis of energy stores, i.e. glycogen and triacylglycerol and also protein. Insulin exerts its effects after binding to a specific transmembrane receptor which possesses tyrosine kinase activity but its precise mechanism of action is unknown.

Glycogen synthesis

Glycogen is stored primarily in liver and muscle and whilst muscle contains a greater total amount of glycogen, higher concentrations are present in liver. The liver is the only tissue capable of donating glucose directly to the circulation and its glycogen content fluctuates throughout a 24-hour period as it serves to top up blood glucose between meals and particularly overnight. After digestion of a meal the hepatic portal vein carries a high concentration of glucose (often in excess of 10 mM) and simultaneously the liver receives newly-secreted insulin from the pancreas by the same route. A raised insulin concentration inhibits glucagon secretion in the pancreas. Thus glucose is converted to glycogen in the liver primarily due to rapid activation of glycogen synthase. This enzyme, which is inactive in the phosphorylated form, is activated by the same phosphatase that acts on phosphorylase **a** and thus activates glycogen synthesis and inhibits glycogenolysis. In the liver the phosphatase forms an inactive complex with phosphorylase **a** but when the glucose concentration rises above 5 mM it (glucose) binds to phosphorylase **a** acting as an intracellular glucose receptor, changing its shape such that it is now susceptible to the action of the phosphatase. Dephosphorylation of active phosphorylase **a** to the inactive **b** form releases the phosphatase which can now activate glycogen synthase. Free glucose in the liver is thus able to stimulate its own conversion to glycogen (Fig. 2.15). Also, the condition of raised insulin and high glucose promotes the synthesis of hepatic glucokinase, ensuring a continued net flux of glucose into liver glycogen.

In muscle, the stimulation of glycogen synthesis by insulin also occurs via a cAMP-independent mechanism and again leads to activation of the phosphatase common to the phosphorylase-synthase system described above. Interestingly, the concentration of insulin required to stimulate glycogenesis is lower in muscle than in liver. Insulin also stimulates the rate of glucose

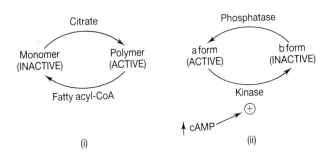

Fig. 2.16 Control of acetyl-CoA carboxylase activity by (i) allosteric effectors and (ii) phosphorylation

transport into muscle and adipose tissue. It has no effect on glucose uptake by the liver where the rate of uptake reflects the glucose concentration gradient across the plasma membrane (i.e. the concentration difference between the blood and the cytosol).

Lipogenesis

The synthesis of fatty acids and their incorporation into their storage form, triacylglycerols, represents a mechanism for conserving the energy of dietary components, fat, carbohydrate and the carbon skeletons of amino acids, which are in excess of the immediate requirements of the body. In addition, the turnover of cell organelles requires the synthesis of phospholipids, glycolipids and sterols, essential components of eukaryotic cellular membranes.

Control of fatty acid synthesis

The rate limiting enzyme of fatty acid synthesis is acetyl-CoA carboxylase, which is under acute control by insulin (stimulatory), and glucagon (inhibitory in liver) and adrenaline (inhibitory in adipose tissue). Like pyruvate dehydrogenase, acetyl-CoA carboxylase is controlled acutely both by phosphorylation and by allosteric effectors (Fig. 2.16). Phosphorylation of the enzyme increases its sensitivity to inhibition by long chain fatty acyl-CoA and decreases its sensitivity to activation by citrate. These methods of control are not mutually exclusive and both act to decrease the activity of the enzyme. Inactivation of acetyl-CoA carboxylase by glucagon and adrenaline occurs via a cAMP-dependent phosphorylation but the rapid activation of the enzyme by insulin which also involves covalent modification is not mediated by cAMP.

The preferred substrate precursors for fatty acid synthesis in the liver are glucose, either from the blood or from endogenous glycogen, and lactate. The supply of acetyl-CoA is ensured by activation of pyruvate dehydrogenase by the raised insulin concentration (Fig. 2.8) and this mitochondrial acetyl-CoA condenses with oxaloacetate to form citrate which overflows into the cytosol. Hence citrate causes activation of acetyl-CoA carboxylase and through the action of citrate lyase provides acetyl-CoA. Provision of pyruvate is ensured

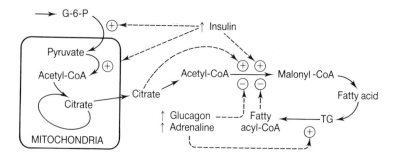

Fig. 2.17 Control of fatty acid synthesis

by an enhanced glycolytic activity due to raised insulin and lowered glucagon levels which give rise to elevated F-6-P and F-2,6-BP concentrations (p. 26). These activate PFK even in the presence of citrate. The overall control of fatty acid synthesis is summarized in Fig. 2.17. Malonyl-CoA has an inhibitory effect on β-oxidation and prevents this pathway from supplying acetyl-CoA and thereby, significant futile cycling.

A more chronic effect of raised insulin is that it leads to an increase in the amount of acetyl-CoA carboxylase enzyme and other key enzymes of the glycolytic and fatty acid synthetic pathways.

Control of triglyceride synthesis

The rate of triglyceride synthesis in both liver and adipose tissue depends mainly on the supply of fatty acyl-CoA. Under anabolic conditions the raised insulin-to-glucagon ratio ensures that triacylglycerol hydrolysis is minimal so that fatty acyl-CoA for triacylglycerol synthesis is derived from lipoprotein-borne lipid (Chapter 8) or from *de novo* synthesis in the tissue. With dietary fat providing in excess of 35% of energy, there is very little new fatty acid synthesis, stored triglyceride being derived from dietary fats. Chronic control of the synthesis of triacylglycerol is exerted through changes in the amount of phosphatidate phosphohydrolase, the enzyme located at the branch point of triacylglycerol and phospholipid synthesis (Fig. 2.18). While the enzyme is always active for basal triacylglycerol synthesis its activity is increased markedly by elevated glucocorticoids.

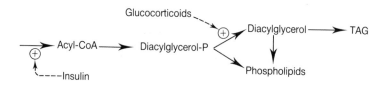

Fig. 2.18 Control of triacylglycerol (TAG) synthesis

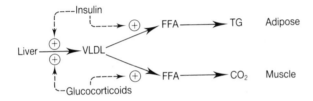

Fig. 2.19 Lipid export from liver

Control of sterol synthesis

The major control point in this pathway is at the level of mevalonate production catalysed by 3-hydroxy-3-methylglutaryl coenzyme-A reductase (HMG-CoA reductase). The enzyme is subject to acute and chronic control which is dealt with in detail in Chapter 8.

Lipid export from the liver

The pathways of triacylglycerol and sterol synthesis converge in the assembly of very low density lipoproteins (VLDL) in the liver (Chapter 8). Synthesis and secretion of this particle are stimulated by insulin and to some extent by raised glucocorticoids both of which increase substrate supply.

The fate of VLDL triacylglycerol depends on the hormonal state of the body (Fig. 2.19). Under anabolic conditions (raised insulin) VLDL-triacylglycerol is hydrolysed by the active adipose tissue lipoprotein lipase (LPL) to provide fatty acids for storage as triacylglycerol. Under stress conditions (catabolic) where glucocorticoids are raised relative to insulin, the VLDL is metabolized preferentially by muscle to provide fatty acids for β-oxidation. The LPL activity of heart and skeletal muscle is increased by stress hormones whilst that of adipose tissue is low under these conditions. The fate of the cholesterylester component of VLDL is described in Chapter 8.

Protein synthesis and turnover

An average adult of 70 kg supports a protein synthesis rate in excess of 400 g per day at an energy cost of 3 kJ/g for peptide bonds. The dietary input of amino acids is approximately 70 g per day and makes a relatively small contribution to the supply created by turnover (Fig. 2.20). Amino acids derived from hydrolysis

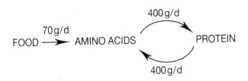

Fig. 2.20 Protein synthesis

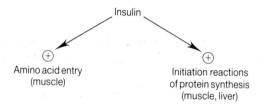

Fig. 2.21 Acute effects of insulin on protein synthesis

of dietary protein are delivered via the hepatic portal vein to the liver where all except branched chain amino acids are incorporated into protein or are catabolized. A raised amino acid level in the circulation, as is seen after a meal, stimulates glucagon release from the α-cells in the pancreas in addition to the glucose-stimulated release of insulin from the β-cells. The increased glucagon stimulates the uptake of amino acids by the liver and allows sufficient gluconeogenesis to prevent insulin-stimulated hypoglycaemia. Thus even in the anabolic fed state some conversion of amino acid to glucose occurs. Insulin also stimulates the uptake of branched chain amino acids into muscle where they are incorporated into protein or transaminated and catabolized.

The precise mechanism by which hormones control protein synthesis in eukaryotic cells is unclear. As stated earlier, in the fed state protein synthesis is stimulated by raised insulin and also by growth hormones when insulin concentrations are high. Protein synthesis is an integral part of gene expression and is controlled predominantly by transcription and the level of messenger RNA (mRNA). Increased transcription produces more t-RNA, ribosomes and mRNA thus providing the necessary components for translation. This process, which is stimulated by both insulin and growth hormone in muscle and liver, is relatively slow compared with acute effects on enzyme activity. Obviously some means of transmitting a signal from the initial peptide hormone–membrane receptor complex must exist but has yet to be elucidated (Chapter 1).

The acute actions of insulin on protein synthesis are two-fold. First, it stimulates amino acid transport into muscle to provide an increased supply of substrate for amino acyl-tRNA formation. Second, it increases polysome number and translation of mRNA into protein in liver and muscle (Fig. 2.21).

3

Energy balance

The concept of nutrient balance introduced in Chapter 2, is of particular importance to the consideration of whole body energy metabolism. In its simplest terms, energy balance can be stated as:

Energy intake − energy expenditure = change in body energy stores

Thus, if intake exceeds expenditure, positive energy balance exists, e.g. growth in children or in the development of obesity. Conversely, when expenditure exceeds intake there is negative energy balance, e.g. starvation, slimming and wasting diseases.

The common observation that most adults maintain a relatively stable body weight (though somewhat less stable body composition – see below) over their adult life is taken as evidence that energy balance must be rather precisely regulated. Such an assumption is strengthened by the fact that if energy intake consistently exceeds energy expenditure by 3 per cent over a period of 10 years, the adipose tissue content of the body would increase by 30–40 kg, increasing body weight by approximately 50 per cent. However, whilst a variety of mechanisms have been identified in the control of energy intake and of energy expenditure, it is still unclear how these are integrated into a regulatory system which monitors and controls body energy content or body weight.

Energy intake

Typical factors involved in controlling energy intake are listed in Table 3.1.

Neural aspects

Early work in experimental animals identified the hypothalamus as important in the control of energy intake. In particular, the ventromedial hypothalamic area was thought to be involved in satiety and the cessation of feeding, whilst the lateral hypothalamic area was more involved in the initiation of eating (i.e. the hunger centre). Whilst these hypothalamic areas are involved in the control of feeding, it is no longer thought that they are controlling *centres* which contain specific nuclei. Furthermore, the few studies undertaken in humans

Table 3.1   Likely factors involved in controlling energy intake in humans

	Factor	Source
Hormonal	Gastrin	Stomach
	Cholecystokinin	Duodenum
	Insulin	Pancreas
	Glucagon	Pancreas
Metabolites	Glycerol	Fat digestion
	Free fatty acids	Fat digestion
	Ketones	Fat metabolism
	Amino acids	Protein digestion
	Glucose	Carbohydrate
Others	Thermogenesis	
	Gastric distension	
	Social influences	
	Food palatability	

failed to show that these hypothalamic areas were as important as in other species, and in primates the limbic system has a role in the control of feeding.

Neurochemistry

A variety of neuropeptides and more classical neurotransmitters have effects on feeding behaviour, and several have been shown to exist within the hypothalamus. Cholecystokinin (CCK) produces satiety in experimental animals, but it is not clear whether the effect is due to CCK released into the blood from the GI tract then having an effect on the brain, or CCK released as a neurotransmitter/neuromodulator within the CNS. Neuropeptide Y (NPY) is present within hypothalamic neurones and does appear to be involved in the initiation of satiety in rats. Furthermore, abnormalities of hypothalamic NPY have been found in genetically obese rats, which are characterized by excessive food intake. Opioid peptides may also be involved in the control of feeding, as the opiate antagonist naloxone induces satiety in both rats and humans.

5-Hydroxytryptamine (5-HT) is involved in the initiation of satiety. This is the focus of substantial research activity at the moment, and a variety of 5HT agonists (e.g. *d*-fenfluramine, fluoxetine) is being used in an attempt to reduce appetite/induce satiety in the treatment of obesity.

Controlling signals

In addition to the importance of specific brain regions and neurotransmitters in the control of food intake, there must be signals from the periphery related to the metabolic state of the body which are involved in the initiation and cessation of feeding. Early theories focused on the maintenance of blood glucose concentration as being of major importance in the control of food intake, and there is no doubt that hunger is a characteristic symptom of hypoglycaemia (i.e. a reduced blood glucose). However, there is less evidence that a high blood glucose (such as during/after a meal) inhibits feeding and other factors are undoubtedly involved. Such factors are likely to include gastrointestinal hormones released during the digestion and absorption of food (e.g. CCK, insulin, glucagon), gastric distension leading to afferent nervous signals passing to the CNS, and changes in the plasma concentration of metabolites such as glycerol, NEFA, ketones and amino acids. In addition, the rise in metabolic rate during and after a meal (the thermic response – see below) may affect body temperature and thus contribute to the control of feeding.

Food intake in humans

In addition to the metabolic/endocrine factors involved in the control of feeding, there are a variety of environmental, social and psychological influences in humans. Thus, the availability of highly palatable foods (usually with a high fat content) frequently leads to over-consumption. There is increasing evidence that carbohydrate intake is one of the main factors sustaining satiety, such that high fat/low carbohydrate foods are associated with a greater overall energy intake to achieve an adequate carbohydrate consumption. In addition, the initiation and termination of eating is very dependent on visual clues relating to the appearance of food and of the amount thought to have been consumed. The complexity of the social and psychological factors affecting food intake is illustrated when one attempts to define the terms hunger, appetite and satiety. *Hunger* is generally regarded as being the desire to eat almost anything. *Appetite* is the desire to eat a specific food – i.e. one may wish to eat one type of food (e.g. chocolate cake) but would rather not eat than consume a different food (e.g. hot dogs). *Satiety* is somewhere between the relief of hunger and the nausea which eventually causes one to stop eating. An example of the imprecise nature of satiety is during holiday/feast periods such as Christmas, Diwali or the end of Ramadan. People can easily consume 2–3 times normal daily energy intake at a single meal and 'feel full', yet when palatable desserts are offered, they still manage to eat more. Other psychological factors, such as stress and depression, can have marked effects on food intake, leading to either undereating or overeating depending on the circumstances and the individual.

Thus, any attempt to modify food intake clinically must address the psychological factors as well as the underlying physiological controllers. It is vital that patients are informed about fat and carbohydrate contents of foods and helped to alter their lifestyle and diets to consume less fat and more carbohydrates. The main benefit to be derived from appetite-suppressing drugs is in helping to achieve such changes.

Energy expenditure

Measurement

For the purposes of this book, the terms *energy expenditure* and *metabolic rate* can be considered as identical, describing the rate of utilization of energy by the

Table 3.2 Methods of indirect calorimetry

Technique	Mouthpiece/nose clip	Cost
Douglas bag	Yes	Low
Respirometer	Yes	Low
Spirometer	Yes	Low
Ventilated canopy	No	Moderate
Respiration chamber	No	High

body. In addition, the term *thermogenesis* (which means heat production) is also used in place of energy expenditure or metabolic rate. However, it would be better to restrict the use of thermogenesis to describe the stimulation of energy expenditure above a basal level, e.g. in response to food, cold or certain drugs and hormones.

For any period in excess of a few minutes, contributions from anaerobic processes are insignificant and so energy expenditure is effectively described by the following equation:

$$\text{Substrate} + \text{Oxygen } (O_2) = \text{Carbon dioxide } (CO_2) + \text{Water} + \text{Energy}$$

The energy released consists of ATP and heat, but as the ATP is utilized so further heat is released. Thus, energy expenditure is also referred to as heat production and provided body heat content (temperature) is constant, this equates to heat loss. Thus, energy expenditure can be assessed by measuring the O_2 uptake and CO_2 production by the body (*indirect calorimetry*) or by measuring heat loss and body temperature (*direct calorimetry*). The latter technique requires extensive, precise measurement facilities (which are extremely expensive) and is inappropriate for most clinical and research purposes. By contrast, indirect calorimetry is less complex and can be fairly inexpensive, requiring gas analysers costing a few thousand pounds as a minimum. Table 3.2 lists the various techniques available for performing indirect calorimetry, the least intrusive to the resting subject and most appropriate for such measurements is the ventilated canopy technique. This is illustrated diagrammatically in Fig. 3.1. Apart from ease of use, the major advantage of indirect calorimetry for measuring energy expenditure is that one can also obtain information on the substrates being utilized. The average amounts of O_2 consumed and CO_2 produced from the oxidation of the major substrates are listed in Table 3.3. With indirect calorimetry, one can measure CO_2 output ($\dot{V}CO_2$) and O_2 consumption ($\dot{V}O_2$) and derive the respiratory exchange ratio (RER), i.e. $\dot{V}CO_2/\dot{V}O_2$. Provided subjects are in steady state with regard to acid–base balance, this RER is equivalent to whole body RQ. Provided urine output is collected to determine nitrogen excretion (allowing the rate of protein oxidation to be calculated) one can determine the rates of fat and carbohydrate oxidation from this RQ value (Fig. 3.2). Furthermore, if the RQ is outside the 'normal' physiological range of 0.71–1.00, and acid base status is stable, one can draw important conclusions

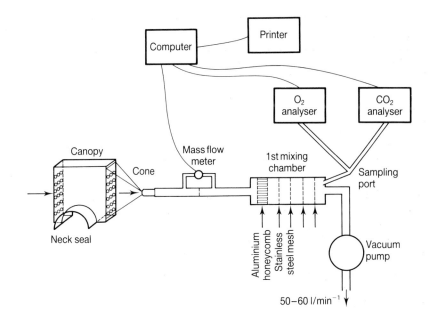

Fig. 3.1 Example of ventilated canopy calorimeter

about the occurrence of *net* ketogenesis (RQ below 0.71, i.e. incomplete oxidation of NEFA) or of *net* lipogenesis (RQ above 1.0, i.e. synthesis of fatty acids from glucose).

Components of energy expenditure

The major components of 24-hour energy expenditure are illustrated in Fig. 3.3. Most adults in the developed world are sedentary, so resting expenditure accounts for at least 60 per cent of the daily total. This resting expenditure can be divided into several constituent parts, basal metabolism, acute effects of food, nutritional status, cold and additional endocrine disease factors.

An alternative way of considering resting energy expenditure is to separate it

Table 3.3 Oxidation of major substrates

Substrate	O_2 used (l/g)	CO_2 produced (l/g)	RQ	Energy yield (kJ/l O_2)
Glucose	0.83	0.83	1.0	21.1
Fat	2.02	1.43	0.71	19.6
Protein	0.97	0.78	0.81	19.3
Ethanol	1.46	0.98	0.67	19.9

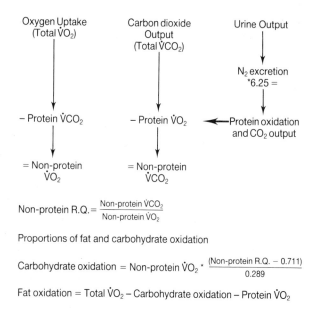

$$\text{Non-protein R.Q.} = \frac{\text{Non-protein } \dot{V}CO_2}{\text{Non-protein } \dot{V}O_2}$$

Proportions of fat and carbohydrate oxidation

$$\text{Carbohydrate oxidation} = \text{Non-protein } \dot{V}O_2 \ast \frac{(\text{Non-protein R.Q.} - 0.711)}{0.289}$$

$$\text{Fat oxidation} = \text{Total } \dot{V}O_2 - \text{Carbohydrate oxidation} - \text{Protein } \dot{V}O_2$$

Fig. 3.2 Estimation of substrate oxidation from gas exchange

into obligatory and facultative components, frequently referred to as obligatory and facultative thermogenesis. The obligatory element represents most of the basal metabolism together with the essential energy expenditure associated with the ingestion, absorption, distribution and storage of food. Thus, obligatory thermogenesis is the sum of the essential metabolic processes. By contrast, facultative thermogenesis is the regulated component of energy expenditure –

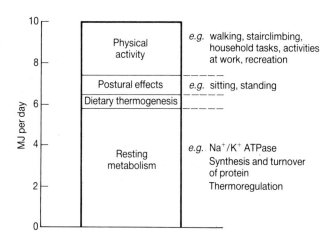

Fig. 3.3 Partitioning of 24hr energy expenditure. Example is for moderately active individual with daily expenditure of 10MJ

the additional effects of food ingestion and the stimulation of metabolism seen with excessive energy intake, cold exposure and the over-secretion of some hormones.

Basal metabolism

In the fasting, resting state the single most important component of energy expenditure concerns the maintenance of ionic equilibrium across cell membranes, in particular the sodium pump (Na^+–$K^+ATPase$). The activity of this pump is not fixed, but can be affected by alterations in thyroid hormone status (increasing as thyroid hormone levels rise). In addition, all of the processes essential for life are energy consuming and contribute to basal metabolism. Examples are cardiorespiratory function, synthesis, degradation and turnover of metabolic intermediates and macromolecules. As might be expected, one of the major determinants of basal metabolism is an individual's total active cell mass, which is directly related to their lean body mass or fat-free mass (see Body composition, below). In addition, age has an influence on basal metabolism, even when expressed in relation to fat-free mass (FFM), with the highest rates of metabolism seen in the first few years of life (up to age 5) and a decline seen with ageing in adults. A major contributor to this is the relative proportions of the vital organs and skeletal muscle in the FFM, with the former having higher rates of metabolism and representing a greater proportion of FFM in infancy. In addition, rates of protein (and other macromolecule) synthesis are highest in early life and decline with ageing. As the rate of protein turnover is usually approximately five times greater than the daily intake, and the energy expenditure in synthesizing peptide bonds is 3 kJ per g synthesized, a protein turnover of 300 g/day in a healthy adult can account for a substantial part of daily resting energy expenditure.

Effects of food

Some of the earliest observations of the stimulation of energy metabolism by food ingestion were made by Rubner, who fed high protein meals to dogs. This led to the term 'Specific Dynamic Effect (or Action)' of feeding and for many years it was thought the effect was specific to protein. However, it is now clear that this is not the case and that in humans, glucose and fat also produce a stimulation of thermogenesis, and in most cases the largest effect is achieved with a mixture of nutrients (i.e. food – see Table 3.4)

The effects of food on energy expenditure can be described as diet-induced (or dietary) thermogenesis, and consist of obligatory and facultative components. The facultative aspects can be reduced by β-adrenoceptor blockade (with drugs such as propranolol) and probably involve activation of the sympathetic nervous system. This facultative component is particularly noticeable when palatable rather than bland meals are consumed, and is greater with high carbohydrate than with high fat foods.

The effects of food on energy expenditure should be considered in two parts, the acute response to a single meal (the thermic response) and the chronic effect of nutritional status (i.e. over- or under-feeding). The thermic response

Table 3.4 Thermic responses to individual nutrients and to food

Nutrient	Thermic response	
	Peak rise in MR (%)	% of ingested energy expended
Glucose	13	5–10
Fat	5	3–5
Protein	25	20–30
Meal*	25	10–15

* The meal contains 50% (energy) carbohydrate, 35% fat, 15% protein

to a meal is affected by meal size, with the magnitude of the stimulation of basal metabolism increasing up to a maximum of approximately 30 per cent, and the duration of the response increasing up to many hours for large meals (Fig. 3.4). Associated with this thermic response are substantial cardiovascular effects; cardiac output can increase by up to 50 per cent and gastrointestinal blood flow remain elevated 2–3-fold for several hours after a large meal. The effect of nutritional status on energy expenditure affects basal metabolism, through alterations in substrate turnover and the hormonal regulators, as well as the response to single meals. Thus, over-feeding in the non-obese is accompanied by an increase in energy expenditure which is less marked in those predisposed to obesity. By contrast, under-feeding is associated with reductions in energy expenditure, not just because the thermic response to food is smaller because less food is eaten, but also because basal metabolism per unit FFM is reduced in under-nutrition.

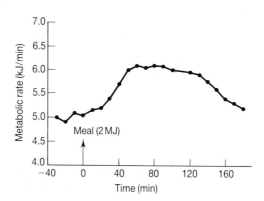

Fig. 3.4 Example of thermic response to food

Effects of cold

Acute cold exposure in adult humans causes an increase in energy expenditure due to shivering. Chronic exposure to cold in many animals species leads to the activation of non-shivering thermogenesis, but there is little evidence that this is important in adult humans. However, babies do have efficient mechanisms of non-shivering thermogenesis (the ability to shiver takes many months to develop) which involve the activation of brown adipose tissue (see below). In adults, mild to moderate cold exposure (insufficient to produce overt shivering) does increase energy expenditure, probably through an increase in muscle tone. Thus, in adult humans the important mechanism of thermogenesis in the cold involves activation of skeletal muscle rather than of brown adipose tissue. This is, of course, much less efficient at generating heat to maintain a normal temperature of the vital organs, as the skeletal muscles are in the periphery and much of the extra heat produced is lost to the environment.

Endocrine factors

Table 3.5 lists the major hormonal effects on energy expenditure. Thyroid status particularly influences basal metabolism and may also act synergistically with the catecholamines. Adrenaline is a particularly potent thermogenic stimulus, the threshold plasma concentration being just above the normal resting plasma adrenaline level. Many factors produce modest increases in plasma adrenaline which have important implications for the stimulation of thermogenesis. The effects of adrenaline are predominantly through activation of β-adrenoceptors, and β-agonists such as isoprenaline are also potent stimuli of thermogenesis. The other counter-regulatory hormones (glucagon and cortisol) stimulate thermogenesis, but are of greater relevance in trauma and injury rather than in the normal state. Insulin should also be considered as a hormone which stimulates energy expenditure, as the synthesis and storage of nutrients which are produced by insulin have an obligatory expenditure of energy associated with them. In addition, high plasma insulin levels may activate the sympathetic nervous system and give rise to catecholamine-stimulated thermogenesis.

Table 3.5 Important thermogenic hormones

Adrenaline
Thyroid hormones
Glucagon
Cortisol
Growth hormone
Insulin (in combination with glucose to stimulate carbohydrate oxidation)

Infection and disease

Many pathological states such as trauma, injury, inflammation, infection, sepsis and certain types of cancer are associated with marked increases in energy expenditure (Chapter 5). Severe burns can cause elevations of resting

Table 3.6 Main components of daily energy expenditure of average weight adults

	Energy expenditure MJ/d	
	Men (75kg)	Women (60kg)
Resting	7.3	5.8
Food	0.7	0.6
Physical activity		
Low	2.0	1.7
High	4.0	3.4

energy expenditure of 70–100 per cent and increases of 10–40 per cent are common in injured or septic patients. In many cases, this stimulation of metabolism arises from the production of cytokines (such as the interleukins and tumour necrosis factor) which act both directly and through activation of catecholamine release.

Physical activity

Details of the increase in energy expenditure which occur with exercise, and the rates of expenditure seen at rest and in various types of activity are given in Chapter 7. Although the potential for increasing total daily energy expenditure is substantial, the sedentary lifestyle of most adults means that activity contributes a modest amount to total daily expenditure (Table 3.6). However, it is now clear that high levels of physical activity have the potential for increasing energy expenditure to a greater extent than the energy cost of the exercise itself. Thus, prolonged high intensity exercise may stimulate energy expenditure for many hours after the activity stops (the excess post-exercise oxygen consumption – EPOC). The mechanisms of this EPOC are unknown, but must include replacement of muscle glycogen stores and repair of muscle damage which may have occurred during the exercise.

Mechanisms of thermogenesis

This section is concerned with possible mechanisms underlying facultative (or adaptive) thermogenesis, and the tissues or organs of the body which may be involved.

Brown adipose tissue (BAT)

This tissue is so-named because of its appearance, the red-brown colouration resulting from its large blood supply and high concentration of cytochromes (components of the electron transport chain). BAT has a much lower triacylglycerol (fat) content and higher cytoplasmic content than white adipose tissue (WAT). In addition, the fat in BAT is contained in several lipid droplets within the cytoplasm whereas WAT has a single lipid droplet occupying most of the volume of each cell. The cytoplasm in BAT contains large numbers of mitochondria which have extensively developed cristae. When lipolysis is stimulated in BAT (usually by the stimulation of β-adrenoceptors by noradrenaline released from sympathetic nerves or by adrenaline or noradrenaline in the blood) the liberation of non-esterified fatty acids (NEFA) within the cells leads to uncoupling of oxidative phosphorylation within these mitochondria. This uncoupling occurs because the NEFA displace the nucleotide guanosine diphosphate (GDP) from a protein thermogenin (which has a molecular weight of 32 000) in the inner mitochondrial membrane, such that the protons (H+) generated during electron transport can re-enter the mitochondrion and be oxidized (releasing heat) without being linked to the synthesis of ATP (Fig. 3.5). Thus, thermogenesis occurs through oxidation of fatty acids without production of ATP.

As mentioned above, BAT is an important site of thermogenesis in neonates (including human babies), some hibernating species and in cold-adapted rodents. There is little evidence that BAT can contribute significantly to whole body thermogenesis in adult humans.

Substrate cycles

There are a number of examples of cycling of substrate which involve the utilization of ATP which leads to the expenditure of energy. The most obvious of such cycles is the fructose-6-P to fructose-1,6-bisphosphate step in glycolysis (Fig. 3.6). Activation of both enzymes involved in forward and reverse reactions will increase ATP utilization without increasing glycolytic flux.

Other examples of such cycling involves the shuttling of substrates between tissues in a series of reactions involving the breakdown and resynthesis of storage materials. Examples of this are muscle glycogenolysis yielding lactate which can then be used for hepatic gluconeogenesis, possibly eventually leading to muscle glycogen resynthesis (an adaptation of the Cori cycle), and the

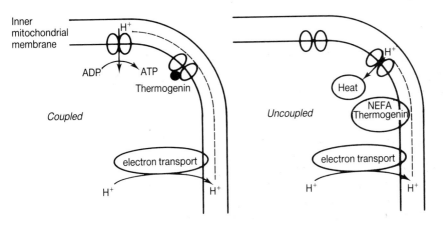

Fig. 3.5 Uncoupling of oxidative phosphorylation in Brown Adipose Tissue

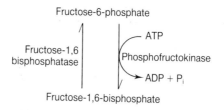

Fig. 3.6 Example of a substrate cycle

triacylglycerol–fatty acid shuttle, whereby adipose tissue lipolysis leads to NEFA release into the circulation; these eventually undergo re-esterification to triacylglycerol in the liver. In the starving state, such triacylglycerol–fatty acid recycling may account for up to 10 per cent of basal metabolic rate, but it is unlikely to contribute more than 1–2 per cent under normal conditions.

Sites of thermogenesis

Obviously, all body tissues have some degree of ongoing metabolism, but it is likely that some are of greater importance than others as sites of regulated thermogenesis. Apart from the BAT mentioned above, it appears that resting skeletal muscle is an important site of thermogenesis, not least because there is so much of it in the normal adult. Approximately, one-third of the thermogenic response to catecholamines seems to be due to increased oxygen consumption in skeletal muscle, but the biochemical basis of this effect is not established.

The splanchnic region (gastrointestinal tract, liver and spleen) has a high rate of energy metabolism and demonstrates a substantial increase in response to catecholamines. A part of this response may be the splanchnic components of the Cori cycle and the triacyglycerol–fatty acid cycle, but there may also be other processes involved.

Body composition

The composition of the body can be considered in gross chemical terms (water, fat, protein, carbohydrate, minerals) or in groupings of similar tissues. The former is illustrated in Table 3.7 for the average weight non-obese individual. Obesity is considered in Chapter 4, but for the present discussion it is sufficient to note that obesity in men exists when body fat content exceeds 28 per cent of body weight, and in women when fat is over 32 per cent of total weight.

As these various components of the body are contained within the cells and organs, a more useful way of dividing the body is into the fat mass and fat free mass (i.e. the chemical fat and the remainder) or into the adipose tissue mass and lean body mass. The adipose tissue mass includes not only the chemical fat (triacylglycerol) but also the connective tissue, cell membranes and cytoplasm within the adipose tissues. Thus, the healthy individual represented in Table 3.7 with 10 kg body fat could actually have approximately 12.5 kg adipose tissue

Table 3.7   Body composition of normal weight adults

	Men		Women	
	Weight (kg)	*%*	*Weight (kg)*	*%*
Protein	11.0	16.0	9.0	15.0
Fat	10.5	14.0	15.0	25.0
Carbohydrate	1.0	1.5	0.9	1.5
Water	44.0	63.5	32.1	53.5
Minerals	3.5	5.0	3.0	5.0
Total	70.0	100.0	60.0	100.0

since the fat content of the tissue is only about 80 per cent of the total mass. From this discussion it should be clear that an individual's lean body mass will be smaller than their fat free mass, and care should be taken when using the terms.

In addition to knowing the weight of the various components of the body, it is also important to be aware of their energy contents. This is illustrated for obese and non-obese in Table 3.8. Consideration of these energy contents makes it rapidly obvious that a substantial, sustained degree of negative energy balance would be needed to return the obese individual to the non-obese state. A negative balance (expenditure greater than intake) of 1000 kcal (4.18 MJ) per day would need to be sustained for 250 days (more than 8 months) to successfully return the patient to the non-obese state. Such a degree of daily negative energy balance is the *most* than can normally be achieved for a sustained period.

Table 3.8   Comparison of body composition in obese and non-obese subjects

	Non-obese		Obese	
	Weight (kg)	*Energy (MJ)*	*Weight (kg)*	*Energy (MJ)*
Protein	11.5	190	12.0	199
Fat	14.0	585	40.0	1671
Carbohydrate	1.0	16	1.0	16
Water	40.5		44.0	
Minerals	3.0		3.0	
Total	70.0	791	100.0	1886

Measurement of body composition

This is extremely difficult to perform accurately in the living subject; some common methods are listed in Table 3.9. Body water content can be estimated

Table 3.9   Some common methods for estimating body composition

Lean body (fat free) mass.
  Total body water – deuterated or tritiated water dilution
  Body cell mass – whole body ^{40}K-counting
  Bioelectrical impedance – estimates volume of conducting material

Body fat
  Skinfold thickness – four standard sub-cutaneous sites
  Imaging – MRI or CAT scanning
  Dual X-ray absorptiometry – low energy X-rays

Both
  Densitometry – underwater weighing or volume displacement
  Anthropometry – no direct information on fatness, but important for assessing size and
              shape

reasonably accurately from isotope dilution techniques, but assumptions have to then be made about the degree of hydration of the fat-free mass in order to estimate the fat content. As fat has a different density (0.9 g/ml) from fat-free mass (usually 1.1 g/ml), if whole body density is measured (by underwater weighing or volume displacement) the fat and fat-free proportions of the body can be estimated. However, the density of fat-free mass is not constant (leading to error), the technique is quite demanding of the subjects, and hence is not widely used.

The potassium content of fat-free mass can be estimated non-invasively by placing a subject in a room screened from external gamma-radiation and using very sensitive counting equipment to determine the body content of ^{40}K. The isotope forms a constant small proportion of total K; however, K concentrations in intracellular fluid are not constant, or the same in everyone, so using the technique to estimate body cell mass does produce errors. Also, 1–2 per cent of total K is extracellular, producing further errors.

Attempts have been made to use imaging techniques (CAT and MRI) to assess total adipose tissue contents of patients, but this would be quite expensive, and undesirable as far as X-ray exposure in CAT is concerned and impractical for many situations. A more promising approach is to use the dual energy X-ray systems involved in assessing bone mineral density to estimate a patient's adipose tissue content, as the X-ray properties of adipose and lean tissues are very different. The X-ray dose with this technique is quite low, and

Table 3.10   Body Mass Index

	Body Mass Index (Weight (kg)/Height^2 (m^2))
Underweight	Less than 20
Normal	20–25
Overweight	25–29.9
Obese	Over 30

the equipment cost is approximately 1 per cent that of CAT or MRI scanners.

The most useful, practically applicable technique for estimating body composition involves simple anthropometry (heights, weights and circumferences), measurement of skinfold thickness, and determination of a subject's bioelectrical impedance. The main information derived from anthropometry is an individual's weight for height. The useful index which best describes this is the Body Mass Index (BMI), which is equal to weight (kg)/height (m)^2. Normal and obese values of BMI are illustrated in Table 3.10. In individual cases the BMI can be misleading, as skeletal frame size (width) has an influence on weight for a given height, and occasionally individuals can be heavy but have a low fat content, i.e. an extensive muscle mass due to physical training such as weightlifting. The most sensible approach to assessing body composition is to combine the measurement of BMI with the determination of the thickness of skinfolds at four standard sites (biceps, triceps, subscapular and suprailiac). The measurements should be made with carefully calibrated spring-loaded calipers by an observer who has been properly trained so that a standard technique is used. In this way, the thickness measured can be used in predictive equations to estimate body density and in turn per cent body fat content.

Bioelectrical impedance analysis (BIA) involves passing very small electrical currents between a hand and foot with surface electrodes and a battery-powered device, and measuring the electrical resistance (or impedance). This is related to the volume of the electrical conductor between the sets of electrodes. Thus, from the measured resistance, and a subject's height and weight, the body water content can be estimated and body fat-free mass and fat mass derived.

On their own, the BMI, skinfold thickness and BIA can produce erroneous estimates of fat mass. However, using all three techniques together allows a more reliable estimate of a subject's fatness to be made.

The other important use of anthropometry is the measurement of circumferences around the waist and hips to estimate fat distribution. Thus, the waist–hip ratio is widely used to characterize fat distribution into a gynoid (female) type when the ratio is low (usually below 0.8) to android (male) type of fat distribution when the ratio is high (usually above 1.0). This has important implications for obesity and its complications, as the metabolic properties of subcutaneous and intra-abdominal adipose tissues differ, with a high waist–hip ratio (more intra-abdominal fat) being accompanied by more complications.

4

Starvation and obesity

The two extreme examples of disturbed energy balance are starvation (negative energy balance) and the development of obesity (positive energy balance). It must be remembered that stable obesity is no longer a state of positive energy balance, the obese individual simply needs a high energy intake to balance their energy expenditure and maintain weight and body composition. The metabolic aspects of starvation and the development and maintenance of obesity will be considered in this chapter. Less severe disturbances will not be discussed, but it should be remembered that in most cases they are less marked examples of the severe alterations in metabolism which are described.

Starvation

The term 'starvation' should be used to describe the situation when no food at all is consumed, but it is frequently used to describe states of severe (but not total) food deprivation. The term fasting is often used interchangeably with starvation, but it is better to consider fasting as something undertaken voluntarily. Starvation and semi-starvation will lead to severe undernutrition in the affected individuals and eventually, of course, lead to death. If there is a shortage of water as well as food, death will occur much faster. The speed with which the undernourished state becomes clinically significant depends on the original body composition and state of health of the individual and the environmental conditions. There are a number of metabolic adaptations to starvation which increase the length of time the starving state can be tolerated, and also some functional consequences of severe undernutrition, both of which will be considered in the following sections. In all cases, it will be assumed that sufficient water is available for drinking.

Body composition

During starvation, the substrates for energy metabolism have to be derived from the body stores. Thus, body composition plays an important role in the events of starvation and the duration for which it can be tolerated. Table 4.1 compares the weight and energy contents of the major body constituents for a normal weight

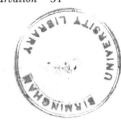

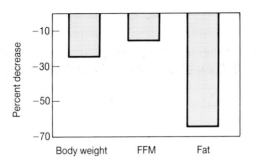

Fig. 4.1 Losses of body weight, fat-free mass (FFM) and fat after 6 months semi-starvation

and an obese individual. As only about one-third of the protein can be utilized (before muscle function is seriously compromized leading to death) it is clear that for a daily energy expenditure of 1600 kcal (6.7 MJ) the non-obese individual's energy stores would last about 75 days. However, such long periods of survival are only possible because of the metabolic adaptations to starvation.

The preferential utilization of the body fat stores was illustrated in an experimental study of semi-starvation (half of normal energy intake for 6 months) performed by Keys and colleagues in the 1940s. As shown in Fig. 4.1, the body fat store was depleted to a much greater extent than the fat-free mass, illustrating the importance of the former in enabling survival. Total starvation will inevitably result in death, which often occurs before the energy stores are completely depleted. For example, the 30 Irish hunger strikers lost 38 per cent of body weight after 70 days of starvation, and by this time 10 of them had died. Severe vitamin deficiencies contribute to the morbidity and mortality of starvation, and infection and disease will speed up the wasting process and hasten death.

Energy metabolism

In the first few days of starvation, there is a rise in resting energy expenditure, probably due to the energy costs of increased gluconeogenesis and ketogenesis.

Table 4.1 Available body energy contents of non-obese and obese subjects during starvation

| | Non-obese | | Obese | |
	Weight (kg)	MJ	Weight (kg)	MJ
Body weight	70.0		100.0	
Protein	6.0	100	6.0	100
Carbohydrate	0.25	4	0.25	4
Fat	11.0	429	35.0	1365
Total		533		1469

As starvation proceeds, resting energy expenditure falls, partly because of the reduction in body weight and fat-free mass, and also because the metabolic rate per unit fat-free mass is reduced. This reduction in resting energy expenditure is partly due to decreases in sympathetic nervous system activity and in plasma free triiodothyronine (T_3) concentrations (see below). In addition to reduced resting energy expenditure, severe undernutrition is accompanied by lethargy and very low levels of spontaneous physical activity so that total daily energy expenditure is decreased substantially. These changes are all of survival benefit, as a reduction in total daily energy expenditure allows body energy stores to last for a longer period of time.

Substrate utilization

Table 4.2 shows the oxygen consumption of the various tissues and organs of a resting, non-obese individual in the normal state. This individual would have a whole-body resting oxygen consumption of about 300 ml/min, which equates to an energy expenditure of about 6 kJ/min. The table also illustrates the different substrates (glucose, fatty acids, ketones) that can be used as fuels for the energy metabolism of the tissues and organs. In the normally fed state, brain metabolism is based exclusively on glucose utilization, with approximately 120 g of glucose being oxidized by the brain per day. During an overnight fast, most of this glucose is provided by mobilization of hepatic glycogen, but approximately 25 per cent is derived from gluconeogenesis. One of the major adaptations to starvation of tissues other than brain is a switch from utilizing glucose as the major fuel to using either fatty acids or ketone bodies. As this adaptation proceeds, the need for glucose diminishes, thus reducing the rate at which body protein is broken down and reducing the amount of energy expended in gluconeogenesis.

Glucose

Plasma glucose concentration falls quickly over the first few days of starvation, falling in normal weight subjects from 5 to 3.5 mM within 3 days, and stabilizes

Table 4.2 Tissue fuel consumption in the 70 kg man (resting)

Tissue	Wet weight (kg)	O_2 consumption (ml/min.)	Fuel*
Skeletal muscle	20–30	70	G,K,F
Adipose	9–13	Small	G,F
Gastrointestinal tract	2.6	58	G,K,F
Blood, etc.	5.5	Small	G
Liver	1.7	75	G,F
Brain	1.5	46	G,K
Lung	1.0	12	G,K,F
Heart	0.3	27	G,K,F
Kidney	0.3	16	G,K,F

* G = glucose, K = ketone bodies, F = fatty acids, not in order of preference.

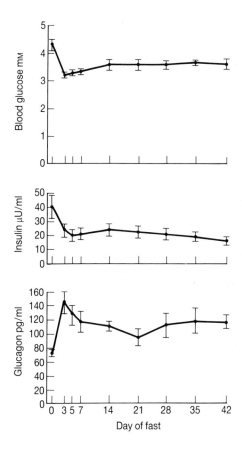

Fig. 4.2 Blood glucose, serum insulin and plasma glucagon response to prolonged starvation. The subjects studied were seven obese volunteers. Values are mean ±SEM. (Reproduced from Marliss *et al.* (1970). *Clin., Invest.,* **49** 2256 by copyright permission of The American Society for Clinical Investigation)

thereafter. This fall in glucose is accompanied by a fall in plasma insulin (to less than 5 mU/l in the non-obese) and a rise in plasma glucagon. Qualitatively similar changes occur during starvation in obese individuals (Fig. 4.2).

In the first few days of starvation, there is still substantial glucose utilization by the brain, the glucose being provided initially from hepatic glycogenolysis followed by hepatic and then renal gluconeogenesis. The substrates for gluconeogenesis are lactate from skeletal muscle glycogen, alanine from muscle protein and glycerol from adipose tissue triacylglycerol (Fig. 4.3), with fatty acid oxidation providing the energy required. Most of the other tissues have markedly reduced rates of glucose utilization, thus sparing glucose for the brain. This reduced glucose utilization is partly due to increased availability and use of fatty acids which reduces pyruvate dehydrogenase complex activity thus decreasing glucose oxidation (the Randle Cycle). The other major factor in reduced glucose oxidation is decreased tissue glucose uptake due to the falls in plasma insulin and glucose which occur in starvation.

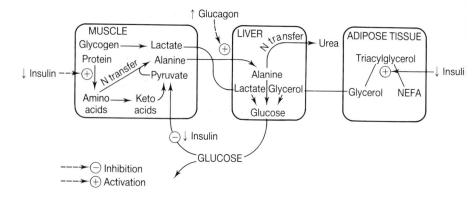

Fig. 4.3 Gluconeogenesis in starvation

Insulin normally inhibits proteolysis, thus the decrease in plasma insulin during starvation allows muscle protein degradation to proceed. With little protein synthesis, this leads to the net loss of amino acids (mainly alanine) from muscle. Increased plasma glucagon stimulates hepatic extraction of alanine from the blood, providing one of the major substrates for the increased rate of gluconeogenesis. By 36 hours of starvation, gluconeogenesis accounts for over 75 per cent of hepatic glucose production, and more than half of the gluconeogenesis occurs via alanine. In starvation, the normal operation of the glucose–alanine cycle (Chapter 2) is interrupted, the muscle amino acids provide both the pyruvate and amino groups for alanine synthesis (Fig. 4.3). Hence, in the early stages of starvation, muscle alanine formation and release correlate well with protein breakdown, but not with muscle glucose utilization. The amino acids most rapidly converted to pyruvate include the branched chain amino acids (except ketogenic leucine). These amino acids can make a net carbon contribution to C_4-intermediates of the citric acid cycle in muscle and can then produce pyruvate via oxaloacetate and phosphoenolpyruvate. The control of this interruption of the glucose–alanine cycle during starvation is not clear but it must include the greatly reduced extraction of blood glucose by muscle resulting from decreased circulating insulin. It is worth noting that the elevated plasma glucagon does not cause mobilization of muscle glycogen glucose which therefore does not provide a source of pyruvate for alanine synthesis.

In summary, as a result of the increasing plasma glucagon concentration and decreasing insulin concentration early in starvation there is a rapid hepatic glycogenolysis together with, and eventually replaced by, glucose provision by hepatic gluconeogenesis from alanine derived from increased muscle proteolysis (Fig. 4.4).

Fatty acids and ketones

The fall in plasma insulin seen with overnight starvation is sufficient to allow the rate of adipose tissue lipolysis to increase (due to the removal of insulin's inhibitory effect) such that non-esterfied fatty acids (NEFA) are released

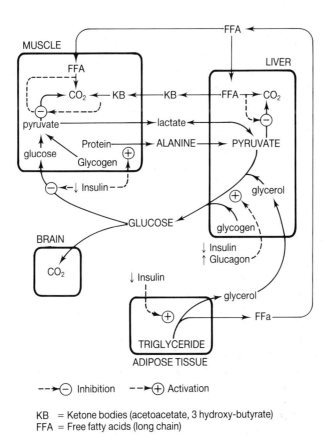

--->(−) Inhibition   --->(+) Activation

KB = Ketone bodies (acetoacetate, 3 hydroxy-butyrate)
FFA = Free fatty acids (long chain)

Fig. 4.4 Glucose sparing for use by brain in the early phase of starvation. KB=ketone bodies (acetoacetate, 3 hydroxy-butyrate). FFA=free fatty acids (long chain)

into the plasma. As starvation proceeds, the rate of lipolysis increases and more NEFA are released. However, the plasma concentration rarely exceeds 2 mM (compared to 0.3 in the fed state), partly because of limited transport capacity (NEFA are bound to plasma albumin) and mainly because the rate of utilization of the NEFA matches their rate of appearance. Some tissues (such as skeletal muscle) use the NEFA as direct substrates for energy metabolism. In addition, the high glucagon:insulin ratio in starvation enables increased hepatic β-oxidation of the fatty acids leading to high rates of ketogenesis. These ketones (acetoacetate and 3-hydroxybutyrate) diffuse into the plasma and distribute throughout body water, making them readily accessible by most tissues. Plasma ketone concentration rises from approximately 0.01 mM in the fed state to 2–3 mM after 3 days of starvation and 5–6 mM after 1–2 weeks, which together with the large volume of distribution of ketones indicates a very high rate of production in prolonged starvation. As well as providing an alternative to glucose, the metabolism of ketone bodies and fatty acids inhibits glucose oxidation in extrahepatic tissues. The increased degree of acetylation of coenzyme A caused by rapid oxidation of ketone bodies and fatty acides increases the proportion of the inactive (phosphorylated) form of pyruvate dehydrogenase, thus preventing irreversible loss of glucose carbon. Any glycolytic breakdown of glucose would thus be channelled to lactate and can be converted to glucose again by hepatic gluconeogenesis. Thus, in starvation, the Cori cycle driven by fatty acid oxidation in liver, is maintained by the glucose sparing actions of fatty acid and ketone body oxidation in muscle. These actions of fatty acids and ketone bodies resulting in the sparing of glucose for brain metabolism during the early phase of starvation are shown in Fig. 4.4.

As adaptation to starvation proceeds, two important factors are the utilization of ketones by brain and the contribution of the kidneys to gluconeogenesis, whereby 50 per cent of total glucose synthesis is renal. These adaptations occur after 4–5 weeks' starvation in obese subjects, at which time total gluconeogenesis has fallen by more than 70 per cent compared to the early stages, with associated reductions in muscle protein breakdown, plasma alanine and urinary nitrogen excretion. The mechanisms underlying the increased oxidation of ketones by the brain are not understood but may involve increased activity (induction) of the enzymes involved in ketone metabolism and improved transport of ketones into the neurones. It is of interest that human neonatal and infant brains, and rodent brains, have a much higher capacity for metabolizing ketones than non-starved adult humans. Fig. 4.5 summarizes the adaptations of substrate utilization during prolonged starvation and illustrates the increased use of ketones by nerve tissue, such that 50 per cent of total brain energy metabolism is derived from ketones after 5–6 weeks' starvation.

Protein

As starvation proceeds, there is a progressive reduction in the rates of protein breakdown and nitrogen excretion. There is a small contribution to this from the fall in plasma free T_3 concentration which occurs in starvation, but the main effect is due to the reduced rates of gluconeogenesis which occur as brain ketone utilization increases. In addition, increased concentrations of ketones in the muscle cells inhibit the oxidation of branched chain amino acids in the muscle cells which reduces the rate of muscle protein breakdown (Fig. 4.6). It is worth noting that this effect is not found in diabetic ketoacidosis, where very high plasma ketone concentrations (over 20 mM) occur at the same time as high rates of muscle protein breakdown.

Hormonal changes

The principal hormonal changes in starvation are a fall in insulin and rise in glucagon. Thyroid hormone production is usually unaffected but peripheral conversion of T_4 to T_3 is reduced (with an increase in reverse T_3 production) contributing to the reductions in resting energy expenditure and protein breakdown seen in prolonged starvation. Starvation and prolonged undernutrition are also accompanied by a reduced activity of the sympathetic nervous system (provided there is not marked fluid loss and large reduction in blood volume) which has important implications for the control of metabolism and which contributes to some of the functional disturbances outlined below. The most

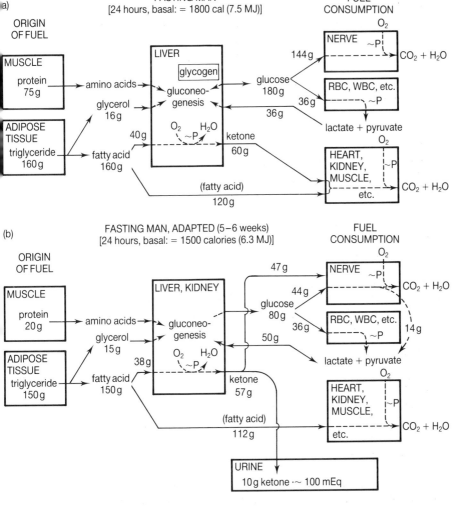

Fig. 4.5 Schematic representation of substrate metabolism in man after a short period of fasting (36hr) (A) and after a prolonged period of fasting (5 to 6 weeks) (B). (Reproduced from Reynold, AC, Stauffacher W and Cahill, G F. The *Metabolic Basis of Inherited Disease* Ed by Stanbury et al, McGraw Hill Book Company, New York)

important effect of reduced sympathetic activity is that lipolysis in adipose tissue does not proceed at an excessive rate. This process is stimulated by the sympathetic nerve supply to the tissue and if sympathetic activity was unaltered, the fall in insulin seen in starvation would give rise to very high rates of lipolysis.

Salt and water metabolism

During the first few days of starvation there is rapid weight loss, not through depletion of body energy stores but because of the loss of 1–2 kg of water from

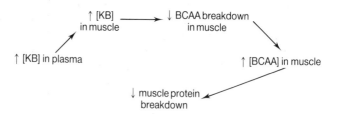

Fig. 4.6 Inhibition of protein breakdown in muscle

the body. Some of this water is extracellular (and accompanied by Na^+ loss) but a substantial proportion is intracellular water associated with the storage of glycogen in muscle and liver. Approximately, 3 g of water are stored with each gram of glycogen, so as the glycogen is broken down as part of glucose production during early starvation, intracellular water is lost as well (together with K^+). This rapid loss of body water in early starvation often has detrimental psychological effects in obese individuals trying to lose weight. If they suddenly reduce their food intake to very low levels, they will lose 1–2 kg (of water) over 3–4 days. However, over the next 3–4 days they will utilize body protein and fat stores (rather than glycogen) as fuels for energy metabolism (and the weight loss will only be 200–300 g).

As starvation proceeds the urinary losses of Na^+, K^+ and nitrogen become markedly reduced. Nitrogen loss in the urine will fall from 12 g/day in the first few days to less than 1 g/day (equated to 6 g body protein) after 5 weeks. Furthermore, whilst in the fed state most nitrogen is excreted as urea, after 5 weeks' of starvation there is virtually no urea output, most nitrogen is excreted as NH_4^+ to preserve acid–base balance in the acidotic state which is characterized by the high plasma ketone levels. In addition, the excretion of NH_4^+ means that other cations (such as Na^+) are retained within the body, conserving extracellular fluid volume.

Functional disturbances

The three major areas of functional disturbance in starvation concern thermoregulation, the cardiovascular system and skeletal muscle. These disturbances can make significant contributions to the morbidity and mortality associated with starvation and severe undernutrition.

Thermoregulation

Control of body temperature in the cold is severely disturbed in starvation and severe undernutrition. In human neonates and infants this is primarily due to atrophy of brown adipose tissue (the main site of cold-induced thermogenesis) and possibly also to a reduction in sympathetic activity. The sympathetic innervation of brown adipose tissue controls its thermogenic function. In the adult human, brown adipose tissue thermogenesis is of minimal importance but starvation and undernutrition still compromise thermoregulation. This is partly due to inadequate peripheral vasoconstriction in the cold, thus failing to reduce heat loss from the body, and partly due to an inadequate thermogenic response. This reduced thermogenesis involves both less shivering and a decrease in non-shivering mechanisms, but the details of the latter are not understood.

Starvation also reduces the ability to sweat and control body temperature in the heat. This is likely to be due to reduced sympathetic activity, as the sweat glands are controlled by the sympathetic nervous system (releasing acetylcholine as the post-ganglionic neurotransmitter), and partly due to reduced body water content and impaired cardiovascular function.

The effects of severe undernutrition on thermoregulation can lead to hypothermia and death in the cold more rapidly than seen in well-nourished people. However, reversal of the undernutrition by feeding leads to normal thermoregulatory function being re-established.

Cardiovascular function

The reduced activity of the sympathetic nervous system and loss of body water and Na^+ in starvation and severe undernutrition have marked effects on the cardiovascular system. Initially there is an increase in resting heart rate which changes to a marked reduction in heart rate after several days. Even in early starvation the maintenance of blood pressure when standing is compromised, and later in starvation it is very difficult for people to maintain an adequate blood pressure when upright. The reduced blood volume and inadequate cardiovascular control mechanisms lead to impaired organ function due to an inadequate blood flow.

Skeletal muscle

One of the first functional changes that can be detected in early starvation and undernutrition is reduced force production by fast twitch muscle fibres. This occurs before many of the classical undernutrition-induced changes in blood chemistry (e.g. fall in plasma albumin or transferrin). As starvation proceeds, obviously loss of muscle bulk provides a more serious impairment of muscle function, eventually leading to breathing difficulties due to reduced respiratory muscle mass. There is also wasting of cardiac muscle which can eventually lead to heart failure.

Pathological aspects of starvation and undernutrition

The most obvious pathological change in severe undernutrition is wasting, especially of the adipose tissue which gives rise to loose skin on the body surface. There is substantial atrophy of the heart and the viscera, but brain size is preserved. Atrophy of the small intestinal mucosa and smooth muscle is particularly noticeable, leading to reduced absorptive capacity which worsens the undernutrition and slows the rate of recovery in re-feeding. Severely undernourished subjects have oedema (especially in peritoneal and pleural cavities) mainly because extracellular fluid volume is better maintained than intracellular volume, so extracellular fluid occupies a larger proportion of tissue volume. The fall in plasma protein contributes to the relatively high extracellular fluid volume.

Starvation ultimately leads to death from a combination of heart failure, vitamin and mineral deficiencies and shortage of metabolic fuel. In starving populations, such as the famines in Africa and Asia, the main causes of death are epidemics of diseases such as cholera and typhoid. These epidemics develop and are so devastating, not because the starving people are particularly susceptible to infection, but because they live in overcrowded insanitary conditions in which the diseases are easily spread.

Summary

The changes in metabolism during starvation illustrate the extent to which adaptive responses occur in an attempt to preserve homoeostasis, minimizing the rate at which body constituents are lost and maximizing survival time. Many of these adaptations occur against a stable hormonal background (low insulin and free T_3 levels, elevated glucagon with plasma corticosteroids and catecholamines little altered), and are predominantly under metabolite-mediated control (e.g. ketone effects on branched chain amino acid use in muscle).

The small changes in the regulatory hormones are critical in determining the extent of protein conservation and thus survival time in starvation. This is clearly illustrated by comparing starvation with uncontrolled Type 1 diabetes mellitus (insulin deficiency) or with major injury/trauma where there are high levels of the catabolic hormones (Table 4.3). It is clear from this comparison that protein loss, electrolyte disturbances and wasting will occur more rapidly in these pathological states than in 'simple starvation'. A more detailed consideration of those other states is presented in later chapters.

Table 4.3 A comparison of metabolic changes in starvation, uncontrolled diabetes mellitus and major injury

	Starvation	*Uncontrolled diabetes*	*Major injury*
Metabolic rate	↓	↑	↑
Energy source	Fat	Fat	Fat
Ketosis	+	+ + +	±
Gluconeogenesis	+ + + then +	+	+ + +
Nitrogen loss	+	+ + +	+ + +
Water/Na$^+$	Initial loss	+ + +	Retention
K$^+$ loss	+	+ +	+ + +

Obesity

Despite the ease with which obese people can be recognized, an exact definition of obesity remains problematic. In general, four possible forms of definition exist:

1. Direct fat measurements: these are based on measurements of body density, total body water content, fall cell mass or total body potassium content.

These techniques are time consuming, expensive and generally limited to research projects.

2. Indirect fat measurements: these are more commonly used and include the assessment of skin fold thickness and the calculation of height/weight ratios (Body Mass Index: BMI). BMI is a mathematical calculation of fat content which was initially developed by Quetelet (Quetelet index) and is calculated from weight (kg)/height (m)^2.

3. Mortality statistics: these are taken from insurance data which allows an ideal body weight for height to be calculated which, in statistical terms, carries no excess mortality risk due to obesity.

4. Visual assessment: this defines only two populations, obese and non-obese, and has little to offer the scientific study of obesity.

None of the methods discussed is without problems; however, the two methods most commonly used in both medical practice and clinical research are BMI and ideal body weight. Using these criteria obesity is defined as a BMI above 30 or a weight 20 per cent or more in excess of ideal body weight. Using these definitions obesity is a common condition with a prevalence in the UK and USA between 10–39 per cent.

Classification of obesity

The classification of obesity is also problematic. More commonly obesity presents as a separate and isolated distinct clinical condition (primary or simple obesity). Occasionally obesity can occur as a consequence of, or in association with, a definable disease or disorder (secondary obesity).

Primary or simple obesity

The vast majority of people who are obese have no demonstrable associated medical condition and are therefore classified as having simple obesity. This term belies the complex nature of primary obesity and hides the fact that the exact aetiology of this condition is unknown. In a majority of people a clear history of caloric excess can be obtained. However, there also appears to be a number of people who remain obese despite apparently moderate caloric intake. It can be argued that in both these situations there is a breakdown in the body's homeostatic mechanisms which normally regulate caloric intake and expenditure.

Secondary obesity

This is traditionally classified as being associated with a congenital syndrome, an underlying endocrine disorder, hypothalamic disease or drug therapy.

Congenital syndromes

Obesity occurs as a feature of a number of rare inherited disorders e.g. Frohlich's syndrome, Alstrom's syndrome, Prader–Willi syndrome and Laurence–Moon–Beidl syndrome. Another common feature of many of these disorders is mental subnormality. Prader–Willi syndrome is of special interest as the obesity in this condition is a consequence of compulsive, uncontrolled eating. The syndrome is caused by a single gene defect on chromosome 15 and this raises the possibility that a protein (the gene product) which regulates eating behaviour may be involved. However, as yet, no gene product or biochemical abnormality has been identified in this syndrome.

These congenital conditions are extremely uncommon and as such are very rare causes of obesity in the general population.

Endocrinological disorders

Obesity is commonly thought of as being a problem caused by 'glands'. In fact the detection of a primary endocrine cause for obesity is extremely unusual. In theory any disruption of the hormonal balance which promotes the action of anabolic hormones or inhibits catabolic hormones will lead to an increased body weight.

Obesity is commonly seen in patients with high systemic concentrations of insulin (hyperinsulinaema), e.g. insulin or sulphonylurea–treated Type 2 diabetics or more rarely in patients with insulinomas. Insulin promotes the storage of triacylglycerols in adipose tissue and glycogen in both liver and muscle. In addition to the increase in adipose tissue mass there is also an increase in lean body mass mediated by the anabolic effect of insulin on protein synthesis. Stein–Leventhal syndrome or polycystic ovary syndrome (PCOS) is a disorder which in endocrinological terms is characterized by high circulating concentrations of the anabolic hormones insulin, oestrogen and testosterone. There is also a marked increase in cortisol metabolism. These hormones predispose the patients with PCOS to obesity and once established the increased adipose tissue mass may exacerbate the hormonal imbalance, promoting continued weight gain.

Alterations in pituitary function can also result in obesity. The presence of an ACTH-secreting tumour in the pituitary gland leads to an increased secretion of the glucocorticosteroid hormone cortisol from the adrenal glands. This condition is called Cushing's disease and is classically associated with marked truncal obesity which characteristically spares the limbs (particularly the legs) This gives the patient with Cushing's disease a distinct appearance which has been described as resembling 'a potato on sticks'.

A reduction in the concentration of catabolic hormones may also lead to an increase in overall body weight. This situation occurs in hypothyroidism where a fall in the concentration of the catabolic hormone thyroxine is often associated with obesity. Hypogonadism in men, with a lowering in the levels of the androgenic and anabolic hormone, testosterone, is also associated with a loss of lean body mass and an increase in adipose tissue which is characteristically deposited in a gynoid distribution.

Recent attention has focused on the possible role of growth hormone in regulating the levels of body fat. Several studies have suggested that the age-related tendency to lose lean body mass and gain adipose tissue reflects a decline in the circulating concentration of growth hormone and insulin like growth factor 1 (somatomedin C). Clarification of the importance of growth hormone in this respect requires further study.

Many of the endocrine disorders discussed are amenable to therapy and appropriate treatment usually leads to an improvement in the level of obesity. However, it should be stressed that primary endocrine disorders are in fact a rare cause of obesity.

Hypothalamic disorders

These condition are extremely uncommon and are only mentioned for the sake of completeness. As previously discussed, eating behaviour appears to be influenced by the hypothalamus and much evidence points to the ventral medial hypothalamus being involved in satiety. If this area is damaged polyphagia and subsequent obesity result. This has been demonstrated in experimental animals and also observed in patients with destructive lesions in this area of the brain. The usual causes of this uncommon condition are trauma, malignancy and infection (TB and syphyllitic granuloma).

Drugs

Some drug therapies, e.g. use of the contraceptive pill (oestrogen) and cortisol therapy, are known to be associated with weight gain. Phenothiazine use can also cause weight gain and this property has been utilized in the treatment of anorexia nervosa. The mechanism by which phenothiazine induces weight gain is probably a combination of appetite stimulation and a reduction in caloric expenditure (reduced basal metabolic rate and physical activity). Recent reports suggest that β-blockers may also cause weight gain, probably via reductions in facultative thermogenesis and physical activity.

Obesity and genetics

Sibling, family and twin studies have implicated a genetic component in the production of the obese state. However, the inheritance pattern is extremely complex and is not compatible with a disorder generated by a simple dominant or recessive gene. It has therefore been suggested that obesity arises as a function of the interaction of multigenes. A comprehensive study of the role of genetics in obesity is severely limited both by its complexity and the undoubted influence of environmental factors.

Obesity and energy intake

A majority of people are obese because of a demonstrable excess energy intake. It is likely that a vast excess of energy intake simply overwhelms the mechanisms that exist for increasing expenditure. If excessive intake is sustained, obesity ensues. The question which this observation raises is, do people who eat themselves into a state of obesity have a disorder in the mechanisms regulating feeding? As previously discussed the regulation of feeding behaviour is complex and as yet ill understood. Neuropeptides appear to be important in the generation of the feeling of satiety and in reducing feeding responses and a number of workers have suggested that a deficiency of neuropeptide Y, in rats, may be implicated in the aetiology of obesity and certain forms of non-insulin dependent diabetes mellitus. However, in man, eating is not a simple, primitive, hypothalamic-initiated and regulated response. There is undoubtedly a cognitive element to eating which allows man to experience both hunger (need for food) and appetite (desire for specific foods). In addition, eating in man is an activity which provides both personal and social rewards.

The familial association of obesity is an indication that in some family groups there is intense pressure to over-eat which may stem from either the need to provide mutual support (mother provides large meals to please family, family eats them to please mother) or as a reaction against more austere times (post-war reaction to rationing). Similarly, in some societies obesity is seen as a reflection of affluence and good health and over-eating is common. It has also been suggested that obesity can be a manifestation of a compulsive personality disorder.

Eating behaviour is clearly influenced by many factors and to demonstrate that obese individuals have abnormal responses to these influences is extremely difficult. However, there have been a number of reports which suggest that the perception of satiety in the obese individual is abnormal. In one study lean and obese individuals were made to draw a fluid meal from a hidden reservoir. Obese individuals consistently felt less satiated, as assessed from psychometric testing, than the lean subjects. In addition the obese individuals drew more fluid per meal from the reservoir than the lean controls. Similar studies have also demonstrated that obese individuals appear to have a reduced ability to adjust their food intake in response to alterations in the caloric value of food. It has been argued that this loss of satiety control may be the result of a hypothalamic abnormality. These studies can however be criticized as they cannot assess whether these individuals are obese as a result of a satiety problem or that feeding problems and dissatisfaction have arisen as a consequence of being obese.

The causes of over-eating are complex but it has been argued that in some people it occurs as a consequence of abnormality in the biochemical mechanisms which induce satiety and reduce the feeding response.

Obesity and energy expenditure

The identification of mechanisms which may be involved in regulating the body's energy expenditure led to the suggestion that a defect in these mechanisms may be involved in the development of obesity. A defect in energy expenditure may be particularly important in those individuals who become obese despite an apparently moderate energy intake.

It was initially suggested that obese subjects have low BMRs and therefore reduced energy requirements. In this situation an intake in excess of these minimal basic requirements, would be stored as fat. However it is now well established that obese individuals actually have higher BMRs than non-obese subjects. This observation has been explained by the finding that lean body mass increases with body weight. Obese individuals therefore tend to have a higher lean body mass than lean subjects. As BMR is a function of lean body mass it is not surprising that this parameter is increased in obesity.

Attention in recent years has focused on the possibility that diet induced thermogenesis (DIT) particularly in brown adipose tissue (BAT), may hold the answer to human obesity. Studies have, however, failed to demonstrate any significant difference in either DIT or BAT in obese subjects when compared to lean controls. In addition the importance of BAT in man has been questioned. BAT is very sparse in adult humans and it has been calculated that BAT metabolism contributes only 1–2 per cent to the total energy expenditure. On the basis of these data it has been suggested that BAT is unlikely to be an important site of DIT in man and therefore has little influence on the regulation of body weight.

DIT may also occur via substrate cycling and it is of some interest that erythrocyte $Na^+/K^+ATPase$ activity appears to be significantly reduced in obese subjects. The interpretation of this data is, however, complicated by the observation that erythrocyte mass is increased in obesity. This suggests that in obesity total $Na^+/K^+ATPase$ activity will be unchanged. In addition, conditions associated with increased weight loss, e.g. hyperthyroidism, do not exhibit changes in the activity of $Na^+/K^+ATPase$.

To date no definitive data has been reported to support the hypothesis that a quantifiable defect in energy expenditure predisposes an individual to obesity. One criticism of all these studies is that the estimates of energy expenditure have been performed in individuals who are obese. It has been argued that in the pre- (or post-) obese state, individuals with a predisposition for obesity may exhibit abnormality in energy expenditure. Some support for this idea comes from the observation that post-obese individuals appear to exhibit both diminished BMRs and DIT responses. Assessment of the importance of this observation must await further study. It is also clear that the pre-obese have difficulties in utilizing dietary fat as fuel for energy metabolism, thus dietary carbohydrate is used at a fast rate (with the fat being stored in adipose tissue) and food intake is stimulated to ensure an adequate supply of carbohydrate.

Obesity and hormones

A number of endocrinological abnormalities are associated with (and undoubtedly result from) simple obesity and their relevance will be briefly discussed. Hyperinsulinaemia is commonly found in obese subjects but in a majority of individuals this resolves completely with weight loss. Thyroid tests need to be interpreted with care in the obese patient. Thyroid function is usually entirely normal in obesity; however, some individuals do show an increase in the concentration of fT_3. This hormone would, in theory, lead to weight loss and the elevated serum concentration in obesity probably reflects increased carbohydrate intake. Obesity is one of the differential diagnoses for Cushing's syndrome (see above). Although obesity is associated with an increase in cortisol production, basal cortisol and cortisol excretion are normal. Dynamic endocrine testing is also normal, with 90 per cent of obese subjects showing suppression of cortisol production on an overnight dexamethasone suppression test. Despite the observation that noradrenaline turnover is reduced in some animal models of obesity, noradrenaline metabolism is normal in human obesity. However, approximately 25 per cent of obese patients have reduced thermogenic responses to infused noradrenaline.

The hypothalamic–pituitary–gonadal axis appears to be normal in obese subjects. Although total testosterone concentrations may be diminished in some obese men this is compensated for by a decline in the concentration of testosterone-binding globulin. These observations are supported by clinical experience which suggests that obese men rarely experience symptoms of testosterone deficiency (gynaecomastia, loss of libido and impotence).

A number of endocrine abnormalities can be demonstrated in simple obesity. However, these abnormalities are invariably reversed when a more appropriate body weight is achieved by dieting. It is therefore generally agreed that these endocrine perturbations are secondary to the obese state and are not implicated in the aetiology of the condition.

Clinical aspects of obesity

Obesity is of clinical interest because it is an extremely common condition (10–39 per cent in USA and UK) and has a significant effect on both mortality and morbidity. Obesity is a condition associated with hypertension, hyperlipidaemia, hyperinsulinaemia and overt diabetes mellitus. All these conditions are independent risk factors for the development of macrovascular disease. It is therefore not surprising that the risk of dying from ischaemic heart disease is extremely high in obese individuals. The development of diabetes mellitus can also diminish the quality of life with the need for regular medication (tablets or insulin) and increased risks of blindness, renal failure and amputations (see Chapter 6; Diabetes mellitus). Obesity can interfere with respiratory function leading to exertional dyspnoea. Patients may also experience sleep apnoea which causes a significant reduction in the concentration of oxygen in the blood. This condition is associated with a poor quality of sleep, morning headaches, increased risk of coronary artery disease and sudden death. If the level of obesity becomes sufficiently gross, the 'Pickwickian syndrome' can develop. This is characterized by obesity, hypersomnolence and apnoea and carries a significant mortality risk.

Digestive complaints, gall stones and osteoarthritis are all more common in obesity. Carcinoma, particularly of the bowel, is also more common in obese individuals and it has been suggested that this may reflect the increased concentration of oestrogen seen in this condition. In addition, gross obesity may diminish the effectiveness of medical therapy, e.g. preventing adequate physical examination, interfering with X-ray investigations, preventing establishment of i.v. access and increasing the risk of anaesthetics. The increased risk of disease and the diminished effectiveness of medical intervention contribute to the significant increase in mortality which is seen in obesity.

Psychological problems are also prevalent in the obese, with depression and neurosis being commonly described. Socially, the obese individual may also experience problems with personal relationships and even find themselves discriminated against in certain jobs. Obesity should never be overlooked as a potential cause or aggravating factor in a patient's illness.

Treatment of the obese patient

The treatment of patients with obesity is often highly unsatisfactory. Currently the only widely used therapeutic option is that of caloric restriction.

Reduction of caloric intake

Dieting is an obvious form of therapy. However, although it may be highly successful in the short term, unless psychological and social problems are also addressed, the rate of relapse is extremely high. Unfortunately, unless a precipitant problem is clearly obvious, the underlying cause of obesity is rarely investigated.

The success of dieting can be improved by a clear explanation of the problem. It should be stressed that although initial weight reduction is rapid the rate of weight loss may then slow down. This is because caloric restriction initially results in the mobilization of hepatic and muscle glycogen. Glycogen has a caloric value of 4 kcal/g but is stored in a complex with water in a ratio of 1:3 (glycogen:water). In contrast, long-term dieting mobilizes triacylglycerols which has a higher caloric value than glycogen (9 kcal/g) and is stored with only a little water. Therefore in the early stages of dieting the expenditure of 1 kcal results in a reduction in body weight of 1 g, while in the later stages of of diet 1 kcal energy expenditure results in only a 0.11 g fall in body weight. In addition, BMR and activity-related energy expenditure tend to fall along with body weight and a reduced energy intake. Exercise, by increasing both BMR and energy expenditure, counteracts the effects of weight reduction on these processes and should therefore form an important part of any weight reduction regime. Dietary instruction and education in 'healthy' eating practices should also form an important part of any diet aimed at achieving long-term weight reduction. In particular diets should be high in complex carbohydrates and low in fat to minimize any problems arising from difficulties in fat oxidation in the obese. Starvation diets are not advocated as they seldom achieve long-term weight loss and can result in hypokalaemia, hypomagnesaemia, hyperuricaemia and gout, ketosis and sudden death.

Surgery

Surgical intervention is considered only in extreme cases of obesity. Operations such a lipectomy, apronectomy, dental splinting, gastric banding and bowel resection all have problems and are seldom a long-term solution to the problem of obesity. Stereotactic neurosurgery directed at ablating the hypothalamic feeding centres has now been largely abandoned.

Drugs

Anorectic drugs which appear to act by increasing adrenergic outflow or by inducing a feeling of satiety have been used in the treatment of obesity with partial success. In many cases the drugs have unwanted and often dangerous side effects. Fenfluramine, a 5HT agonist, has been used to induce a state of satiety and a reduction in food intake. However, side effects which included nausea, diarrhoea, excessive dreaming, and the precipitation of severe depression on abrupt withdrawal severely limited its use. Recently, dexfenfluramine has been introduced and although this drug acts in a similar manner to fenfluramine it is reported to have fewer side effects. Research continues into developing a therapeutic agent, perhaps based on specific regulatory neuropeptides, which can be safely used to modify feeding behaviour.

Amphetamine and amphetamine-like drugs stimulate adrenergic hormone release which increases BMR and induces an exaggerated DIT response. Their use has been shown to result in significant weight loss. However, the side effects of addiction and the precipitation of acute psychotic states has led to these drugs being largely abandoned. Thyroxine also increases BMR and can induce weight loss and lower serum lipids; however, the use of thyroxine as a dietary aid has not been generally endorsed as it has been shown to cause mobilization of lean body mass, have a detrimental effect on bone calcification and can, at high doses be cardiotoxic. During the second World War it was noted that some workers in munitions factories became hypermetabolic and suffered a large weight loss. Investigation showed the increase in thermogenesis to be mediated by a compound called dinitrophenol (DNP). DNP has subsequently been shown to be a mitochondrial uncoupler and act in a similar way to the thermogenin protein found in the mitochondria of BAT. Although this compound did find its way into some slimming preparations the high incidence of side effects led to its use being banned. Currently the search for safe pharmacological agents which induce thermogenesis in obese subjects continues.

Despite the problems listed the future looks encouraging for physicians caring for patients suffering from obesity. An increased understanding of the regulation of normal body weight and the possible defects which occur in obesity may point the way to specific therapies. Currently the development of drugs to modify eating behaviour or thermogenic responses seem promising. The definitive treatment of obesity may, however, come from a completely different area of medical research. Patients with certain cancers often experience a large loss in weight which is unrelated to caloric intake or tumour mass. It has been shown that these tumours produce a compound, now called cachexin, which mediates this rapid decline in body weight. The possibility that this or a similar compound could be used in the treatment of obesity is currently being investigated. However, any treatment for obesity will be successful only if combined with a programme of nutritional education of the patient to ensure their previous eating behaviour and food choice is changed. Without such actions, any drug treatment will be associated with a return to the obese state when the treatment ends.

5

Trauma

An understanding of the metabolic basis of trauma was hindered for centuries by the continued practice of the ideas of Hippocrates and Galen that health could be regained by restoring the imbalance in the four body humors, phlegm, blood, yellow bile and black bile, by purging, starvation, bleeding, cupping and even fever therapy. Such treatment which involved vomitting, diarrhoea and sweating was entirely inappropriate and in many cases it was the treatment itself rather than the disease or trauma which killed the patient. The Irish physician Robert Graves, better known for his description of exophthalmic goitre, however found that mortality from typhus fever was reduced dramatically when patients were given food and drink. This apparently simple treatment of 'feeding the fever' was quite revolutionary.

By the first quarter of the 20th century it was apparent that fever was accompanied by an increased metabolic rate and negative nitrogen balance which could be ameliorated to some extent by nutritional support. As improved nursing care, particularly in prevention of infection, led to increased patient survival a gradual understanding of the chronic metabolic consequences of trauma emerged. The metabolic pattern seen in fever was mirrored in major illness or injury and exacerbated when infection was also present and Cuthbertson in a study of long bone fractures described distinct stages in the metabolic response to injury. An immediate shock or ebb phase of up to 24 hours, where cellular activity is depressed is followed by a hypermetabolic or flow phase which may last for weeks depending on the severity of the injury. Finally, a restorative anabolic phase, during which tissue is repaired and lean body mass lost in the ebb phase is replaced, leads to a full recovery of the patient.

In some ways the metabolic consequences of severe injury resemble starvation in terms of increased protein catabolism and leads to loss of lean body mass. Indeed, the protein catabolism of trauma is exacerbated by starvation, inability to eat or lack of appetite. The injured tissue itself acts like a separate organ and makes extra metabolic demands on the patient, as does the rise in body temperature which is a feature of the hypermetabolic phase. Basal metabolic rate will increase approximately 15% for every degree centigrade rise in body temperature. It is thus not surprising that common features of major illness are fatigue and weight loss, the weight loss occurring much faster in trauma than during starvation.

Injury such as long bone fractures of the leg causes both neuroendocrine and humoral responses (Fig. 5.1) Signals from the site of injury reach the brain via afferent sensory pathways and the spinal column signalling the release of adrenaline from the adrenal medulla and a number of hypothalamic hormone-releasing factors which act on the pituitary. This effect can be prevented by the use of a spinal block. A number of cytokines are also released from the site of injury. These have both local and more generalized actions including actions on the thermoregulatory centre in the hypothalmus.

The initial shock or ebb phase

The metabolic response of an animal under threat or stress is to prepare itself for 'fight or flight'. Even in the absence of injury this involves the release of adrenaline stored in the adrenal medulla with the consequent elevation of blood pressure and heart rate and the mobilization of readily metabolizable substrates from tissue stores. This defence response is seen in some patients about to undergo surgery even before administration of the anaesthetic and is compounded by neuroendocrine responses of the surgical insult or injury itself which initiates a barrage of stimuli focused mainly on the hypothalamus and hind brain. The

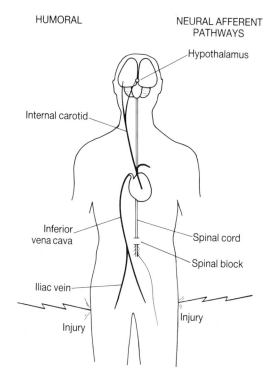

Fig. 5.1 Neuroendocrine and humoral responses to tissue injury

release of hormone-releasing factors from the hypothalamus in turn stimulates the pituitary to release ACTH, prolactin, growth hormone and oxytocin.

The immediate metabolic changes of the ebb phase are thus due to a sympathetic response leading to release of catecholamines. There is often a decreased cellular vitality during this phase associated with loss of blood or plasma from the wound and a decreased oxygen supply to peripheral tissues as the body routes blood to vital organs. However, although there is often a decreased energy expenditure associated with a decrease in body temperature, the body as a whole prepares itself for the subsequent hypermetabolic phase by the general mobilization of energy-providing substrates. The neuroendocrine response in the pancreas causes a rise in glucagon secretion. The body is thus switched to a catabolic mode and serum concentrations of glucose from liver, lactate from muscles and free fatty acids from adipose tissue rise (Fig. 5.2). A glucose tolerance test performed 6 hours after severe trauma shows no, or only a slight, insulin response. The raised free fatty acid concentration and the release of cortisol and growth hormone, will also antagonize the action of any circulating insulin. Thus at a time when plasma glucose concentration rises the ability of insulin-sensitive tissues, particularly muscle and adipose tissue, to clear glucose is severely reduced due to an insulin lack. Consequently there is an increased utilization of free fatty acids as respiratory substrate and, in the absence of insulin, hepatic ketogenesis is increased.

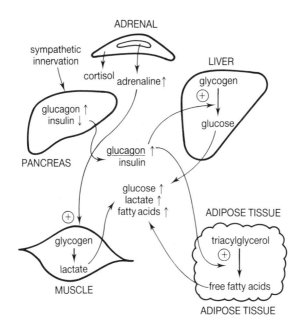

Fig. 5.2 Metabolic response of the ebb phase

The hypermetabolic or flow phase

The short period of decreased energy expenditure is followed by a hyper-metabolic phase which may last for several weeks despite visual healing of wounds. The magnitude of the metabolic changes in this phase reflects the severity of the trauma.

The phase is characterized by increases in heat production (body tempera-ture), resting metabolic expenditure, respiration and pulse rate (Table 5.1). These increases are further accentuated in burned patients, where there is often considerable evaporative heat loss, and in cases of infection. A healthy individual at rest for instance consumes approximately 25 kcal/kg/day and increases this by about 20 per cent if allowed to walk freely (Table 5.2). To maintain zero energy balance an energy intake of between 20 and 30 per cent greater than the measured metabolic energy expenditure is required since such an individual utilizes food inefficiently. After minor surgery resting metabolic expenditure is increased by about 10 per cent, after multiple fractures by 20 per cent. This may increase to 50 per cent on infection such as in peritonitis and to as much as 100 per cent with extensive burns.

The metabolic demands on the traumatized patient may thus be very high and the observation of Hippocrates that those who are fat around the belly best survive disease was very astute. Fat is indeed the major respiratory substrate throughout the hypermetabolic phase, irrespective of the severity of trauma. Of major concern clinically however is the negative nitrogen balance due to the rapid loss of skeletal muscle protein. Protein loss is greater in the well-nourished

---

Table 5.1   Physiological features of the flow phase

1. Increased heat production (body temperature).
2. Increased resting metabolic expenditure.
3. Increased respiration rate.
4. Increased pulse rate.

Table 5.2   Effect of injury on resting metabolic expenditure

Healthy individual at rest	25 kcal/kg
Healthy individual + walking	+20%
Uncomplicated surgery, e.g. vagotomy	+10%
Multiple fractures	+10–20%
Major surgery + sepsis, e.g. peritonitis	+25–50%
Major burns	+50–100%

Figures quoted as % healthy individual at rest.

young patient than in the poorly nourished elderly. An understanding of why this occurs and how to restrict or even eventually prevent it will be of great value in the management of the traumatized patient. The general metabolic response to the flow phase is shown in Fig. 5.3.

Glucose metabolism

The increased circulating concentration of glucose may be a teleologically determined response to satisfy the requirements of damaged tissues. Such tissues have an obligatory requirement for glucose which is metabolized anaerobically, probably by macrophages and cells of the immune system and glucose utilization may be 4-fold greater than in corresponding undamaged tissue. This of course is very wasteful in terms of energy yield since although ATP may be generated locally by anaerobic glycolysis the conversion of the end product of this pathway, lactate, to glucose by hepatic gluconeogenesis requires twice as much ATP as is generated in the damaged tissue. The raised concentrations of catabolic hormones associated with stress, catecholamines, glucagon, cortisol and growth hormone, may also be an adaptive response to stimulate hepatic gluconeogenesis and continue the provision of glucose from the other major substrates for gluconeogenesis, glucogenic amino acids and in particular alanine, released from muscle. In general the rise in blood glucose

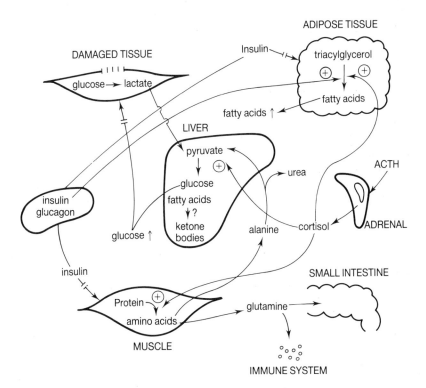

Fig. 5.3 Metabolic response during the flow phase

concentration reflects the severity of the injury but the high rate of metabolism is a wasteful process delaying recovery.

The initial suppression of insulin secretion seen in the ebb phase is followed by a period of insulin resistance in the flow phase. While insulin secretion by the pancreatic β-cells returns to normal or even exceeds normal, the insulin concentration is inappropriately low for the prevailing raised glucose concentration of the flow phase. The resistance of peripheral tissues to insulin is probably due to the antagonistic actions of cortisol and growth hormone and the raised circulating concentration of free fatty acids. A glucose tolerance test at this stage is again abnormal and resembles that of the non-insulin dependent diabetic patient, i.e. lowered tolerance and reduced rate of glucose clearance.

Protein metabolism

Of particular importance in the flow phase is the loss of lean body mass. The negative nitrogen balance is due to loss of protein nitrogen from skeletal muscle brought about by a disturbance in the homoeostatic balance between muscle protein synthesis and degradation as a result of insulin resistance and raised cortisol levels. During moderate to severe trauma there is decreased protein synthesis while protein degradation is unchanged. In sepsis and severe trauma protein synthesis is again decreased while protein degradation is increased leading to rapid loss of protein. In such cases nitrogen balance is not restored in the early stages of the flow phase, even in well nourished patients given adequate nutritional support. This breakdown of muscle proteins yields essential amino acids for protein synthesis in the liver but the muscle itself appears to catabolize branched chain amino acids preferentially, transaminating the nitrogen to pyruvate or glutamate. The plasma concentrations of all amino acids are raised during the flow phase but alanine and glutamine are particularly high. Alanine serves as a carrier to the liver of waste nitrogen for urea synthesis and the minimum three-carbon requirement for gluconeogenesis, processes which are stimulated by the essentially catabolic hormone mode of the body. The rationale for a raised glutamine concentration is unclear but may relate to the increased requirement of this amino acid by rapidly dividing cells. *In vitro* experiments suggest that glutamine is involved in muscle protein balance and stimulates protein synthesis. It accounts for approximately half of the intracellular free amino acid pool of muscle and in trauma, where there is net protein breakdown, glutamine is lost from the muscle due possibly to some change in the regulation of the glutamine transport system and thus the intracellular concentration falls. Glutamine is virtually an 'essential' amino acid for rapidly dividing cells such as the enterocyte of the small intestine (Fig. 5.4) and extra demands are made after trauma due to the cells involved in the tissue repair processes. This demand is increased further if infection is associated with the injury as cells of the immune response divide rapidly. Glutamine may serve as an energy source in such cells as well as providing essential nitrogen for the synthesis of purines and pyrimidines of DNA and RNA. Under normal conditions dietary glutamine is probably all consumed by the enterocytes and thus the glutamine for lymphocytes and other dividing cells is derived from muscle. In trauma or infection the glutamine content of muscle may decrease by as much as 50 per

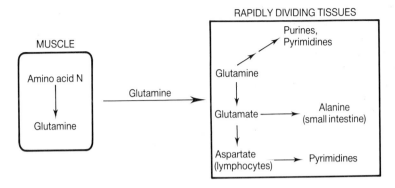

Fig. 5.4 Utilization of glutamine by rapidly dividing tissues (small intestine, lymphocytes)

cent as the body seeks to satisfy the demands of tissue repair and lymphocyte proliferation where glutamine utilization may increase up to 4-fold. There is also a marked increase in glutamine consumption by the GI tract (up to 14 g per day) and kidney (4 g per day) during stress and particularly when nutrition is difficult this glutamine must come from the body's protein store, muscle.

Besides the specific roles of alanine and glutamine, amino acids are also required by the liver for the synthesis of plasma proteins to replace those which may be lost at the site of injury. Local humoral responses to injury and to infection are responsible for inflammation and the production of cytokines such as interleukin-1 (IL-1), interleukin-6 (IL-6), leukaemia inhibitory factor (LIF) and tumour necrosis factor (TNF) by the endothelium, macrophages and lymphocytes (Fig. 5.5). IL-1 and TNF have local actions on vascular tissue. Both are procoagulants and cause vascular congestion leading to reduced blood flow and accumulation of leukocytes and platelets at the site of endothelial damage. Besides such local actions these cytokines generate a systemic response including the stimulation of hepatic gene expression for the acute phase proteins, anti-proteases, haptoglobin, complement proteins, fibrinogen, cerulosplasmin, ferritin, C-reactive protein, acid α-1 glycoprotein and serum amyloid A. Again when nutrition is a problem, amino acids for the synthesis of these proteins will be supplied by the muscle. The cytokines also suppress the synthesis of several 'household' proteins such as lipoprotein lipase, albumin and cytochrome P_{450} and thus severe injury with sepsis may result in altered lipid and drug metabolism (Table 5.3).

Fat metabolism

Although protein breakdown is increased to provide substrates for gluconeogenesis it does not become the major source of energy for the body as a whole even after severe injury. As stated earlier, damaged tissue has an almost obligatory requirement for glucose, obtaining the bulk of its energy from glycolysis. However, studies on resting metabolic expenditure and nitrogen balance in patients who had undergone a variety of surgical operations suggested that even in cases where nitrogen excretion was greatly increased, e.g. massive soft tissue injury, protein contributed only 20–25 per cent of total calories. Even under

Table 5.3   Protein synthesis changes in the flow phase

A. *Increased synthesis (hepatic acute phase proteins)*
Antiproteases, haptoglobin, complement proteins, fibrinogen, ceruloplasmin, ferritin, C-reactive protein, acid α-1 glycoprotein, serum amyloid A.

B. *Decreased synthesis*
Lipoprotein lipase, albumin, cytochrome P_{450}.

these extreme catabolic conditions, as in starvation, body fat was still the major endogenous energy source. The increase in serum free fatty acid concentration of the flow phase is proportional to the severity of the injury, and because of the associated insulin resistance of this phase many tissues continue to use free fatty acid as respiratory substrate despite the high carbohydrate load. Fat administered intravenously, as Intralipid for instance, is cleared more rapidly in the hypercatabolic state and mobilization of triglyceride from adipose tissue is not inhibited by the existing hyperglycaemia, raised insulin concentration or by glucose intake as it is in the fasting patient.

In starvation, where increased mobilization of fat also occurs, hepatic ketogenesis yields alternative oxidizable substrates to glucose, that is aceto-acetate and 3-hydroxybutyrate, to satisfy the energy requirements of muscle and brain (see Chapter 2). It might be expected that raised ketone body levels would also be a feature of the flow phase of injury but this does not seem necessarily

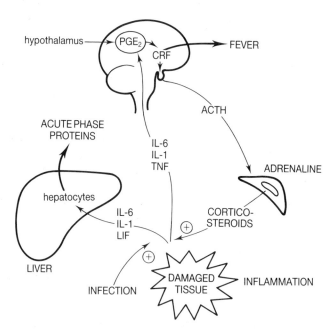

Fig. 5.5 Simplified cytokine response to local tissue damage

to be the case. Some studies have reported no or only a slight rise in ketone body levels following trauma while others have described an appreciable rise. It may be that the variable response relates to the sensitivity of ketogenesis to the prevailing insulin concentration. Whereas the concentration of insulin might be too low to overcome peripheral resistance it may be high enough to inhibit ketogenesis. However, even in cases where ketone body concentrations rise following trauma, unlike in starvation, this is insufficient to compensate for non-utilization of glucose and is unable to prevent continued muscle protein breakdown and gluconeogenesis.

Increased heat production

A further component of the flow phase of severe injury and especially with associated sepsis is a rise in body temperature. Some microbes and toxins are intrinsically pyrogenic but usually the febrile state is due to the action of endogenous pyrogens such as the cytokines interleukin-1 and interleukin-6, tumour necrosis factor and interferons. Localized cutaneous inflammation serves to elevate the local temperature, causing an increased blood flow to carry inflammatory cells to the site of injury to attack any invading organisms and increase the metabolic activity of these cells. Cytokines produced by the endothelium, lymphocytes and macrophages also have autocrine activity and stimulate their own production. For instance, IL-1 and TNF are potent stimulators of IL-6 gene expression and protein synthesis. As described earlier, these have important vascular and haemostatic actions. However, the cytokines also have important metabolic consequences for the whole body (Fig. 5.5). They are carried in the blood to the liver, where they induce the acute phase response described above, and to the brain, exerting an action on the preoptic area and anterior hypothalamus, possibly via prostaglandins and cyclic AMP to raise the thermoregulatory set point by inhibiting the firing rate of warm-sensitive neurones. Given such a response the question arises as to whether fever is beneficial. Much of the evidence in favour has again come from *in vitro* studies. Certainly local production of cytokines increases leukocyte accumulation at the site of damage and bacterial infection and would thus help contain the spread of infection by increasing the activity of phagocytic leukocytes.

In general a moderate rise in body temperature may have an overall beneficial effect on immunological defence mechanisms by enhancing the processes involved in initial antigen recognition and subsequent metabolism. However, there is as yet no direct link between this and a more favourable outcome from infection, although a marked rise in body temperature would have a deleterious effect on these same processes.

Nutrition and recovery

Nutritional support of the traumatized patient must take into account the extra energy demands and marked nitrogen loss of the flow phase. The nutritional state of the patient before injury is also important since malnourished individuals have little labile protein available for catabolism in the flow phase and may be unable to survive even a moderate weight loss. Further, immobility in patients confined to bed causes atrophy of skeletal muscle and contributes to a negative nitrogen balance. Nitrogen loss as a result of depletion of muscle protein is maximal between 4 and 8 days after simple injury, such as long bone fracture, and is usually less than 60–70 g. In more severe cases which may involve secondary infection, for example major thermal burns, the total nitrogen loss may exceed 300 g and of course loss of such an enormous amount of lean body mass may be critical.

Bulk calories may be provided as carbohydrate and fat to meet the estimated energy requirement, and raising the ambient temperature and excluding infection may decrease this by lessening the thermogenic stimulus. In general nutritional support during injury ameliorates to some extent the metabolic response to injury and has a positive effect on nitrogen balance. However, the problem of rapid nitrogen loss remains. Attempts to prevent this have included increasing dramatically nitrogen intake but this proved no better than diets with an adequate energy intake. Similarly branched chain amino acid (BCAA)-enriched diets have been used on the premise that they stimulate the biosynthesis and diminish the degradation of protein in animal muscle *in vitro*. However, such diets failed to prevent the decrease in skeletal muscle protein synthesis and the negative nitrogen balance in patients undergoing elective cholecystectomy.

Glutamine supplementation on the other hand may have a definite beneficial effect. The observation that muscle protein synthesis is directly related to muscle glutamine concentration and that muscle glutamine falls dramatically after injury suggests that intracellular glutamine promotes conservation of muscle protein. The amino acid itself is unstable in aqueous solution but stable in short chain peptides which on infusion into humans are hydrolysed into their constituent amino acids. Supplementation of parenteral diets with alanyl–glutamine greatly improved the nitrogen balance of patients undergoing major surgery (elective resection of carcinoma of the colon or rectum). Moreover, the intramuscular glutamine concentration remained close to the preoperative value through the flow period and such treatment represents a promising approach. What will be important is whether an improvement in nitrogen balance is of clinical benefit to the patient.

The return to homoeostasis may be a prolonged process as the body slowly adapts to the changing metabolic demands brought about by the injury. A gradual understanding of these changes has enabled improved management of the patient during the ebb and flow phases, particularly through nutritional support. This has been aided by the development of the naso-gastric tube and also by improved dietary formulations which can be given parenterally. Thus diets may be tailor-made for specific patients and the dangers of over- or under-feeding and perhaps misfeeding may be obviated. Such specific nutritional support is critical in helping patients through the hypermetabolic phase and preparing them for the anabolic phase during which lean body mass is replaced.

6

Diabetes mellitus

Diabetes mellitus is a disease which was first recognized by the ancient Greeks. The term diabetes means siphon and refers to the observation that patients with diabetes produce large quantities of urine. The term mellitus (meaning honeyed) was added later and reflects the observation that the urine of patients with diabetes mellitus is sweet. We now know that both the diuresis and sweet-tasting urine are caused by the presence of glycosuria. The fact that diabetes could take several clinical forms was also acknowledged by the early physicians. Descriptions of a wasting disease associated with thirst, polyuria and early death clearly refer to insulin dependent diabetes mellitus. In contrast, a condition associated with corpulence and stupor was also recognized and this would be compatible with the classic description of non-insulin dependent diabetes mellitus.

Since the introduction of insulin in the 1920s, deaths from acute diabetic emergencies have become rare and most diabetics are able to live relatively normal lives. However, as the life expectancy of diabetic patients increased it became apparent that the long-term complications of diabetes have a significant effect on the overall mortality and morbidity of the disease. Diabetes mellitus is a common condition with an incidence in the general population of 1–5 per cent. The treatment of diabetes and its complications therefore has a major impact on society both in human terms and on the allocation and cost of health care resources.

Definition, diagnosis and classification

Diabetes mellitus is a metabolic disorder which occurs as a consequence of insulin deficiency or increased peripheral insulin resistance. The classical biochemical abnormality of untreated diabetes mellitus is an uncontrolled rise in the serum concentration of glucose which is usually accompanied by glycosuria. The reduced effectiveness (or absence) of insulin also produces a series of metabolic abnormalities which results in diabetes being associated with elevated serum lipids, accelerated platelet aggregation and an increase in thrombotic tendency.

The World Health Organisation (WHO) have laid down strict criteria for the diagnosis of diabetes mellitus (Table 6.1). An individual with a fasting glucose above 7.9 mM or a random glucose of 11.1 mM, by definition, has diabetes mellitus. There is, however, 'a grey area' between individuals who have normal glucose tolerance and those with overt diabetes mellitus. Individuals with fasting glucose levels between 6.7 mM and 7.9 mM or with a random glucose measurement between 7.9 mM and 11.1 mM are said to be glucose intolerant. The significance of this diagnosis will be discussed later. In some cases a formal glucose tolerance test (GTT) may be needed to firmly establish the diagnosis of diabetes mellitus as distinct from glucose intolerance. Currently, the standard GTT requires that the patient is starved overnight and then receives 75 g of glucose orally. Blood glucose measurements are made before and 2 hours after drinking the glucose. The interpretation of data from a GTT are as described for starved and random tests (see above and Fig. 6.1). The WHO has also classified diabetes into six types (Table 6.2) according to aetiology; however, this discussion will be restricted to insulin dependent diabetes, non-insulin dependent diabetes and glucose intolerance.

Aetiology of diabetes mellitus

Insulin dependent diabetes (Type I)

Insulin dependent diabetes mellitus (IDDM) is a state of insulin deficiency which usually occurs as a consequence of pancreatic β-cell destruction. It is thought that an individual may possess a genetic predisposition to the development of IDDM. Insulin dependent diabetes has a strong association with the HLA haplotype B8;DR4 and a negative association with HLA B7 and DR2. The HLA haplotype B8;DR4 is commonly found in a number of organ-specific autoimmune diseases which is taken as strong circumstantial evidence that IDDM is an autoimmune disease. It is argued that when susceptible individuals are exposed to an environmental toxin (e.g. viral infection or chemical β-cell toxins) some degree of pancreatic damage occurs, releasing pancreatic antigens which initiate an autoimmune reaction resulting in inappropriate and unregulated β-cell destruction. If a sufficient mass of β-cells is destroyed the development of insulin dependent diabetes is inevitable. Support for a humoral autoimmune process in the development of IDDM comes from the

Table 6.1   WHO criteria for the diagnosis of diabetes mellitus using a 75g oral glucose tolerance test. Data refers to capillary whole blood

	Fasting glucose (mmols/l)	Glucose (mmols/l) 2 hrs after OGTT
Non-diabetic	Less than 6.7 mmol/l)	Less than 7.8 mmols/l
Impaired glucose tolerance (IGT)	Less than 6.7 mmols/l)	7.8 to 11.1 mmols/l
Diabetes mellitus	Greater than 6.7 mmols/l)	Greater than 11.1 mmols/l

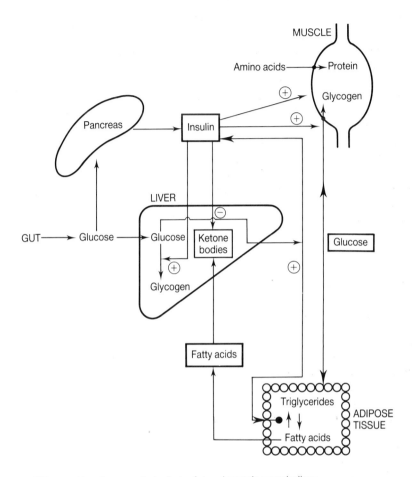

Fig. 6.1 Effects of insulin on carbohydrate, fat and protein metabolism

observations that some patients with insulin dependent diabetes have antibodies directed against islet cells, insulin or C-peptide in their serum. These antibodies are often present at high titre just prior to or just after the development of overt diabetes. It should be noted, however, that only 50 per cent of insulin dependent diabetics ever have anti-islet antibodies. Similarly, although the presence of these antibodies suggests that an individual may develop diabetes, anti-islet antibodies are not a totally reliable predictor of disease. Further data implicating an autoimmune aetiology for IDDM comes from animal studies which have shown that the pancreases from animals who are developing diabetes are heavily infiltrated with activated T-lymphocytes. It has also been shown that during active isletitis, β-cells uncharacteristically express class 2 HLA antigens (D-antigens). These data have been taken as evidence that the β-cells may have been infected and transformed by virus(es), stimulating the expression of inappropriate antigens, initiating a self-perpetuating cycle of cell destruction. These data also suggest that the autoimmune destruction of the pancreas is mediated predominantly by T-lymphocytes and that the development of

Table 6.2   Classification of diabetes and probable mechanisms by which diabetes is generated

Classification of diabetes	Mechanism for diabetes
Insulin dependent/type 1	Insulin deficiency
Non-insulin dependent/type 2	Relative insulin deficiency – peripheral insulin resistance
Gestational-diabetes (GDM)	Increased insulin resistance
Secondary diabetes due to endocrine disease	Increase in antagonistic hormones. e.g. thyrotoxicosis
Pancreatic disease	Relative to absolute insulin deficiency
Malnutrition related diabetes (MRDM)	Relative to absolute insulin deficiency
Diabetes secondary to drugs	Impaired insulin secretion or increased insulin resistance
Maturity onset diabetes of the young (MODY)	Relative insulin deficiency

specific antibodies may be a secondary phenomenon. It is now recognized that a long prodromal phase can occur between the initial pancreatic insult and the development of diabetes. This presumably reflects the available β-cell mass, the rate of β-cell destruction, and possibly the severity and frequency of the environmental challenge. During this prodromal phase individuals can often be shown to have islet and insulin antibodies and abnormalities of insulin dynamics as assessed during a standard glucose tolerance test. However, the use of such tests in the screening for early diabetes is still in question.

Non-insulin dependent diabetes (Type II)

Non-insulin dependent diabetes mellitus (NIDDM) is a heterogeneous disorder which probably includes conditions with a variety of abnormalities in insulin release and action. It has been argued that NIDDM (Type II A) is a condition characterized by delayed or reduced secretion of insulin in response to physiological stimulation. These patients tend to be phenotypically more like IDDM patients (younger and thin) than the classical obese patient with NIDDM. There is also a syndrome of maturity onset diabetes of the young (MODY) which, as the name suggests, is the syndrome of NIDDM occurring in a young person. The exact aetiology of this condition remains unresolved but the clustering of cases in families suggests that there is a strong genetic element to the disease. Patients with classical NIDDM (Type II B) tend to be older and are often obese. In these patients the circulating insulin concentration is often normal or elevated when compared to the levels found in non-diabetic individuals. This relative hyperinsulinaemia suggests that these patients are insulin resistant rather than insulin deficient. The exact mechanism of this insulin resistance is unknown but theoretically could include a reduction in the number of functional insulin receptors, a decrease in the affinity of existing receptors for insulin or a post-receptor defect which interferes with the generation and/or propagation of the insulin second messenger. It is probable that examples of all these abnormalities exist but patients with NIDDM are rarely investigated in such detail. As with MODY there appears to be a strong genetic element in the development of NIDDM and in some families the inheritance pattern of NIDDM is consistent with an autosomally dominant condition.

Glucose intolerance

This is diagnosed on the basis of data obtained from an oral glucose tolerance test. The condition is not an absolute marker for the development of overt diabetes mellitus. In fact if individuals with glucose intolerance are retested 5 years after initial diagnosis only 15 per cent have developed diabetes while a further 15 per cent will have a 'normal' test. This means 70 per cent of these individuals continue to have glucose intolerance, and may have an increased risk of developing hypertension and macrovascular disease (see p. 87, Chronic complications of diabetes).

Metabolic actions of insulin

Insulin is a peptide hormone produced by the β-cells of the pancreas. It is an anabolic hormone which stimulates the formation of metabolic storage compounds such as glycogen and triacylglycerols. Insulin also activates the glucose transporter in muscle and adipose tissue which increases the supply of glucose to these metabolically active tissues.

Insulin secretion is stimulated *in vivo* by the presence of glucose, or an insulin secretion promoting gut peptide, in the portal circulation. Insulin, at high concentration, reaches the liver where it stimulates the metabolism of glucose via glycolysis and the Krebs cycle. Surplus glucose is converted into the storage compound glycogen. Hepatic glycogen is extremely metabolically active and 80–90 per cent of this store is mobilized during overnight fast. In the face of a large supply of dietary fuels and high concentrations of insulin the hepatic catabolic reactions of gluconeogenesis, β-oxidation and ketoneogenesis are inhibited. Insulin clearly acts on hepatic metabolism to stimulate the synthesis of metabolic stores and regulate the supply of fuels, such as glucose, into the systemic circulation. The liver also inactivates 80 per cent of the insulin within the portal circulation. Therefore, under normal conditions, the concentration of insulin in the systemic circulation is normally considerably lower than that found in the portal system.

In the systemic circulation the primary sites of insulin action are the skeletal muscle and adipose tissue. Insulin activates the insulin sensitive glucose transporter in both these tissues, which results in an increased rate of glucose uptake and an increased supply of metabolic substrate. In skeletal muscle the increased supply of glucose and the elevated concentration of insulin promotes the accumulation of glycogen. This is achieved by the coordinated activation of glycogen synthesis (via allosteric and covalent modification of glycogen synthetase) and inhibition of glycogenolysis (via phosphorylation of phosphorylase and phosphorylase kinase). Skeletal muscle glycogen is mobilized considerably more slowly than hepatic reserves and is therefore an important metabolic store which is used during extended fast (days). Insulin also stimulates glycolysis and the tricarboxylic acid (TCA) cycle thereby increasing energy availability to the working muscles. In addition to its metabolic function insulin also promotes amino acid uptake and protein accumulation in skeletal muscle (by inhibiting proteolysis).

In adipose tissue an increased supply of glucose and the presence of insulin can stimulate fatty acid synthetase leading to the formation of fatty acids. However, this is only of quantitative importance in humans when carbohydrate intake exceeds total daily energy expenditure. Activation of glycolysis in adipose tissue by insulin provides energy and glycerol for triacylglycerol re-esterification. It is likely that insulin's most important effect in adipose tissue is to inhibit lipolysis which combines with the stimulation of re-esterification to increase fat storage. When needed, the stored triacylglycerol in adipose tissue can be mobilized to supply fatty acids which are metabolized via β-oxidation to yield energy and acetyl-CoA.

It is clear that insulin is primarily an anabolic hormone which regulates the supply of glucose into the systemic circulation, facilitates the synthesis of energy stores in the form of glycogen, triacylglycerols and promotes protein deposition.

Biochemistry of diabetes mellitus: acute presentations

The pathophysiological consequences of acute insulin deficiency can be predicted from the previous discussion (Fig 6.2). The partition between portal and systemic glucose concentrations is removed and therefore all the dietary-derived glucose moves directly into the systemic circulation causing significant hyperglycaemia. In the absence of insulin, hepatic metabolism swings in favour of gluconeogenesis and glycogenolysis. Glucose derived from both these processes is released directly into the systemic circulation making a major contribution to the hyperglycaemic state. In addition the reduced rate of glucose uptake by adipose tissue and muscle makes a small but significant contribution to the overall hyperglycaemic state. The presence of significant endogenous glucose synthesis and reduced glucose utilization explains why diabetic patients remain hyperglycaemic even during a starvation diet (which prior to the 1920s remained the mainstay of therapy). The presence of high glucose concentrations in the blood has a number of physiological sequelae. Glucose is normally reabsorbed by the proximal renal tubule but once the capacity of glucose reabsorption is exceeded, glucose escapes into the urine. The presence of glucose in the loop of Henle and distal tubule acts as an osmotic diuretic resulting in the production of large quantities of dilute urine (polyuria). As a consequence of this increased urine production the tubular transit time of the urine shortens dramatically, decreasing the ability of the kidney to reabsorb water. The accumulated effects of these processes can result in such a dramatic diuresis that severe dehydration occurs. Dehydration and increasing serum osmolarity activates the hypothalamic thirst centre, promoting a marked drinking response (polydipsia). If the level of dehydration cannot be adequately compensated, intravascular volume depletion, hypotension and reduced peripheral circulation result. Inadequate perfusion reduces tissue oxygen supply which leads to increased anaerobic metabolism, lactic acid formation and creation of a metabolic acidosis.

The systemic insulin deficiency promotes glycogenolysis and muscle catabolism with the production of gluconeogenic substrates such as pyruvate, lactate and alanine which are released into the circulation. In adipose tissue, lipid breakdown results in a rise in the serum concentration of triacylglycerols, free fatty acids and glycerol. The presence of free fatty acids in the serum promotes insulin resistance, thereby exacerbating the state of insulin deficiency. Gluconeogenic precursors and fatty acids are transported to the liver and in the absence of insulin the former are used to synthesize glucose. The synthesis of glucose is clearly inappropriate and its release into the circulation serves to perpetuate the hyperglycaemic state. Fatty acids undergo unregulated β-oxidation producing concentrations of acetyl-CoA which exceed the capacity of the normal routes of metabolism (via Krebs cycle) and thus lead to the production of ketone bodies (see Chapter 2). Ketones are released into the circulation and make a significant contribution to the worsening metabolic acidosis. At this point the condition of diabetic ketoacidosis (DKA) exists (see Fig 6.3).

The presence of a metabolic acidosis promotes the efflux of K^+ from cells (via a K^+/H^+ exchange) to preserve acid–base balance. Much of the potassium is

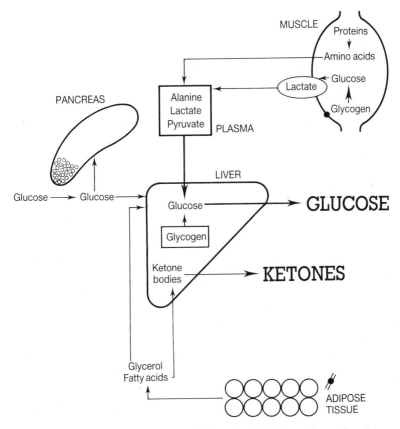

Fig. 6.2 Effects of insulin deficiency on metabolism of carbohydrates, fats and protein

lost as a result of the severe diuresis and depletion of the total body potassium pool ensues. However, the rapid efflux of potassium from the tissues into the serum can, paradoxically, lead to potentially dangerous hyperkalaemia. In an attempt to compensate for the metabolic acidosis respiratory drive may be increased, leading to a pattern of breathing known as Kussmal breathing (described as air hunger) which is characteristic of DKA. In addition, the metabolic acidosis also reduces myocardial efficiency and increases the risk of life-threatening arrhythmias.

It is clear that in the absence of insulin many of the pathological changes described are self-perpetuating and unless the patient is treated they will continue to deteriorate, proceeding to a state of coma and eventually death. This description of the biochemical abnormalities which occur in diabetic ketoacidosis emphasizes the important interaction of metabolic pathways and the impact of disordered metabolism on physiological functions.

In non-insulin dependent diabetes or the early stages of insulin dependent diabetes (pre-ketotic) where the biochemical abnormality is a relative insulin deficiency or systemic insulin resistance, hepatic function remains relatively normal. The ketogenic pathway is very sensitive to insulin and the presence of even low concentrations of insulin in the portal blood are sufficient to inhibit ketogenesis thereby protecting the patient from ketoacidosis (i.e. NIDDM patients do not develop ketosis). The abnormalities in metabolism

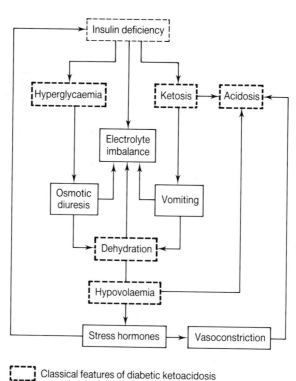

┌─ ─ ─┐ Classical features of diabetic ketoacidosis
└─ ─ ─┘

Fig. 6.3 Pathophysiology of insulin deficiency

in this situation are therefore chiefly confined to hyperglycaemia and lipid abnormalities (hypertriglyceridaemia and hyperlipidaemia). As the condition can sometimes go undetected for relatively long periods of time, serum glucose concentrations can often climb to very high levels (> 40 mM). Despite the lack of ketoacidosis these patients are still at great risk from severe dehydration, increased serum osmolarity and a marked increase in the risk of developing a major venous thrombosis. If untreated these patients also proceed to coma and death. This condition is termed Diabetic Hyperglycaemic Hyperosmolar Non-ketotic Coma. The clinical signs and biochemical abnormalities with their underlying causes are summarised in Tables 6.3 and 6.4.

Table 6.3 Biochemical signs and their causes in diabetes mellitus

Biochemical signs	Cause
1. Hyperglycaemia	(i) Decreased uptake of glucose by peripheral tissues. (ii) Increased hepatic glycogen mobilization. (iii) Increased hepatic gluconeogenesis.
2. Glycosuria	Glucose load exceeds capacity for reabsorption in renal tube.
3. Ketoacidosis	Increased β-oxidation of adipose tissue derived fatty acids in liver. Leads to raised hepatic acetyl CoA concentration and ketone body synthesis.
4. Ketonuria	Ketone load exceeds capacity for reabsorption in renal tubule.
5. Hyperlactataemia	Mobilization and metabolism of muscle glycogen to lactate: Lactate released as precursor of gluconeogenesis (Cori cycle).
6. Hyperlipidaemia	Free fatty acids derived from increased lipolysis in adipose tissue.
7. Hypertriglyceridaemia	Increased synthesis of triacylglycerol in liver and increased VLDL synthesis.
8. Hypovolaemia/ Hyperosmolarity	Excessive loss of body water as urine due to glucose acting as an osmotic diuretic.
9. Hyponatraemia	Loss of body sodium as a result of glucose-induced osmotic diuresis.

Chronic complications of diabetes

Since the instigation of insulin therapy there has been a dramatic improvement in life expectancy of patients with diabetes. However, it has become apparent that even treated diabetes is associated with a number of life-threatening chronic complications. The high incidence of macrovascular disease in long-standing diabetes suggests that the condition is associated with widespread and accelerated atherosclerosis. Disorders of the microvasculature result in diabetic nephropathy and retinopathy while degeneration in nerve

Table 6.4   Clinical symptoms and their causes in diabetes mellitus

Symptoms	Cause
1. Polyuria (nocturia)	Retention of glucose in renal tubule as glucose load exceeds the absorptive capacity. Glucose acts as an osmotic diuretic causing the production of large volumes of urine.
2. Thirst	CNS driven response to dehydration. May be mediated by angiotensin produced in response to hypovolaemia.
3. Polyphagia	Hunger stimulated by non-utilization of dietary glucose.
4. Weight Loss	Increased catabolism of all metabolic fuel stores – muscle glycogen and protein and adipose tissue triacylglycerol.
5. Tiredness	Muscular weakness due to (i) proteolysis and mobilization of muscle protein (ii) reduced availability of metabolic substrate (glucose).
6. Blurred vision	Systemic dehydration of the lens, aqueous and vitreous humor reducing visual acuity.
7. Vomiting	CNS driven response to ketones stimulating the area postrema in the floor of the fourth ventricle.
8. Hyperventilation (Kussmaul breathing)	Respiratory compensation to metabolic acidosis (raised lactate and keto acids in plasma).
9. Itching	

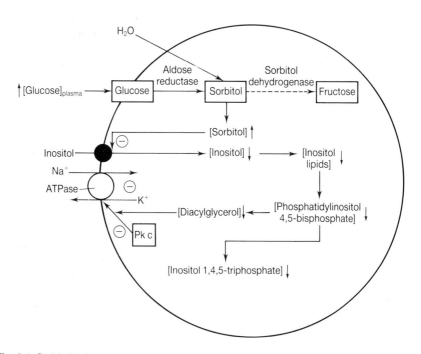

Fig. 6.4 Sorbitol/polyol theory

function accounts for the various forms of diabetic neuropathy (somatic and autonomic). The exact aetiology of diabetic complications remains unknown but it has been suggested that a single biochemical abnormality may underlie them all. Although far from proven, one attractive hypothesis is termed the polyol theory. This broadly states that in insulin insensitive tissues, hyperglycaemia drives the synthesis and accumulation of intracellular sorbitol. Sorbitol accumulation may be associated with intracellular inositol depletion which is thought to modify the activity of membrane-bound $Na^+/K^+ATPase$. This theory is particularly attractive as it incorporates abnormalities in both inositol (or its derivatives) and $Na^+/K^+ATPase$ and both these compounds are known to function as regulators of cell function (see Chapter 1).

Treatment of diabetes mellitus

Acute disturbances

Diabetic ketoacidosis

In diabetic ketoacidosis the two biochemical abnormalities which require urgent treatment are dehydration and insulin deficiency. The total fluid deficit can be in excess of 5 litres and this should be replaced over 6–8 hours. Fluid is usually given as 0.9 per cent (w/v) saline. However, severe hypotension may require administration of colloid to effect a more efficient expansion of the intravascular volume. In older patients, or those known to have cardiac problems, careful attention to cardiovascular status is necessary and may require the use of a central venous pressure line (CVP). Careful monitoring of serum potassium is also mandatory and it should be remembered that, regardless of the serum potassium concentration determined on initial measurement, the patient is potassium depleted. All fluids should have potassium supplementation which should be altered in accord with changes in plasma concentrations. Insulin therapy is required for two reasons, firstly to reduce the plasma glucose concentration but more importantly it inhibits the synthesis and facilitates the metabolism of ketone bodies. Normoglycaemia is often achieved before full correction of the ketoacidosis. In this situation the patient requires continued insulin therapy but in order to prevent hypoglycaemia, glucose (as 5 per cent dextrose) may need to be administered with the insulin.

The metabolic acidosis rarely requires therapy in its own right and is usually corrected when the patient is rehydrated. Occasionally sodium bicarbonate is used (severe acidosis, severe intravascular fluid depletion or myocardial impairment) but should always be administered with potassium supplementation (hypokalaemia can result from rapid correction of the acidosis) and with regard to limiting large swings in osmolarity and pH which might cause cerebral oedema.

Diabetic hyperosmolar hyperglycaemic non-ketotic coma

The major abnormality in this condition is dehydration and this needs to be treated aggressively with fluid replacement. Fluid is usually given in the form of 0.9 per cent sodium chloride. Occasionally, however, the osmolarity of the serum is so high that half normal saline or even 5 per cent dextrose may be preferred. Fluid balance and cardiovascular status should be monitored and this may require a CVP line. Insulin requirements are often small and care should be taken to avoid rapid reduction in serum glucose concentrations as this can be accompanied by cerebral oedema. Temporary anticoagulation, unless indicated for associated conditions, e.g. myocardial infarction, has largely been discontinued.

Long-term therapy

Diet

Diet remains an important form of therapy for diabetes mellitus. The diet is designed to facilitate the control of blood sugar but in appropriate patients (obese non-insulin dependent or severe glucose intolerant patients) may effect a cure. It is now recognized that the correct diet may reduce the incidence of the macrovascular complications in diabetes. In 1982 the British Diabetic Association produced a set of dietary recommendations which have been widely adopted. These state that the diet should be composed of 50–60 per cent complex carbohydrate, 30 per cent fat (predominantly in the unsaturated form), 15 per cent protein and 30–60 g of fibre. Energy restriction is incorporated as appropriate. This diet is designed to reduce glucose absorption, minimize atherogenic potential and to protect renal function. These suggestions are the basis of any 'healthy diet' and the general population should probably be encouraged to adopt similar eating patterns. Consequently, the concept of a specific diabetic diet is gradually being replaced by the idea that diabetics should be encouraged to watch energy intake and eat a healthy low fat, high carbohydrate diet.

Oral hypoglycaemic agents

These agents fall into two groups; the sulphonylureas and biguanides. Metformin is the only drug from the biguanide group in use in the UK. This drug inhibits hepatic gluconeogensis and may also have a direct stimulatory effect on the insulin receptor. Metformin does not stimulate insulin secretion and does not therefore exacerbate hyperinsulinaemia. This has two beneficial effects: it reduces the tendency of the patient to gain weight and there is a very low incidence of hypoglycaemic reactions associated with its use. It is not surprising that the main indication for the use of metformin is in obese diabetic patients. Its use, however, is restricted by the relatively low patient acceptability (nausea) and the contraindications in patients with renal, cardiac or respiratory disease where there is a significant risk of inducing lactic acidosis.

Sulphonylureas have been widely used as oral hypoglycaemic agents since they were introduced in the 1940s. Their mode of action is complex and includes direct stimulation of insulin secretion and increased peripheral utilization of glucose. The effect on insulin secretion means that these drugs do exacerbate hyperinsulinaemia and are consequently associated with weight gain and hypoglycaemia. Recently, the problem of hypoglycaemia has become increasingly recognized and a number of sulphonylureas are being abandoned because of this problem (chlorpropramide and glibenclamide).

Insulins

Insulin was first used in clinical practice in 1921. This followed its discovery and partial purification from the pancreatic islets of laboratory dogs. Commercially-produced insulin was initially obtained from the pancreas of cows (bovine) and more recently from pigs (porcine). This cross species use of insulin has been possible because insulin has a highly conserved primary peptide structure with only one amino acid change between the human and procine hormone. Over the last few years human insulin has become widely available. Human insulin was initially made via the chemical modification of porcine insulin. More recently the functional human insulin gene has been inserted into *E.coli* which then synthesize and secrete human insulin. There is no evidence to suggest that the use of human, as opposed to porcine, insulin confers any clinical benefit; however, human insulin is now in common usage. The indications for the use of insulin in the treatment of diabetes are not always clear-cut. Obviously, a patient with insulin dependent diabetes who has had an episode of ketosis needs life-long insulin therapy. However, many patients are placed on insulin to simply improve their glycaemic control or in an attempt to reduce the risk of developing diabetic complications. These patients do not have an absolute requirement for insulin and its use requires careful consideration of the benefits versus the risks of treatment. Hypoglycaemia is the most feared and potentially most dangerous complication associated with insulin therapy. Patients and the relatives of patients receiving insulin should be instructed in the recognition and treatment of hypoglycaemia. Insulin therapy is usually given by subcutaneous injection and it is worth pointing out that this mode of administration creates an abnormal distribution of insulin in the body. In a normal individual portal insulin concentrations are high, in order to effect changes in hepatic metabolism, whilst the concentration of insulin in the systemic circulation is low. In contrast, subcutaneous insulin administration results in very high systemic insulin concentrations and it has been argued that this hyperinsulinaemia may aggravate the tendency of diabetics to develop both atherosclerosis and hypertension. In addition hyperinsulinaemia dramatically increases the patient's tendency to gain weight. This can promote insulin resistance, increasing the individual's insulin requirement and exacerbating the tendency for weight gain. This clearly creates a very undesirable 'vicious cycle' which can be broken only by restriction of both insulin and energy intake.

Treatment of diabetic complications

The treatment of established complications is dictated by the clinical situation and in most instances diabetic patients are treated in an identical manner to similarly affected patients without diabetes. Peripheral vascular and coronary artery surgery, renal dialysis and renal transplant surgery are increasingly offered to appropriate patients, irrespective of their underlying diabetes. It is still apparent, however, that diabetic complications have a significant effect on overall mortality. Deaths are usually attributable to macrovascular disease (particularly in the non-insulin dependent patients) and renal failure (particularly the insulin dependent patients).

Attention has recently been focused on the possibility of identifying and treating factors, other than glycaemic control, which might influence the development of diabetic complications. The two advances in this field are the treatment of serum lipid abnormalities and systemic hypertension.

Diabetes is classically associated with hypertriglyceridaemia, which has been suggested to be an independent risk factor for the development of atherosclerotic macrovascular disease. Currently, diabetologists are studying the effects of early treatment of this lipid abnormality with dietary manipulation and drug therapy (usually fibrates) where appropriate.

The association of diabetes and essential hypertension has generated considerable interest in both the world of diabetes and cardiology. It has been suggested that hyperinsulinaemia and insulin resistance could be a mechanism by which hypertension develops and influences the development of atherosclerosis. This might explain the high incidence of hypertension in the diabetic population. It has also been shown that hypertension accelerates the development and progression of a number of diabetic complications. Hypertension is a major risk factor in the development of macrovascular disease which has been identified as an important cause of death in diabetic patients. In addition, recent studies have shown that the development and progression of diabetic renal disease to end stage renal failure is directly related to the degree of systemic hypertension. Currently all diabetics are regularly assessed for the presence of hypertension (defined as a blood pressure of 140/90 or higher) which is treated aggressively with hypotensive drugs. Although not universally accepted, there is growing evidence that angiotensin converting enzyme inhibitors should be the first-line antihypertensive drugs in diabetic patients.

Diabetics are known to be prone to macrovascular disease and it has been shown in a number of trials that there is an increased tendency for thrombosis in diabetic patients. The demonstration of the effect of aspirin therapy in acute myocardial infarction has led to the suggestion that diabetics should receive low dose prophylactic aspirin therapy.

The true evaluation of all these treatments awaits the results of well controlled, long-term clinical studies.

7

Homoeostasis and metabolic control during exercise

Muscle tissue accounts for about 30 per cent of the body mass, perhaps 20 kg in an average man. Despite its bulk the contribution of muscle to the total resting metabolic rate is small because its resting metabolic rate is very low. However, muscle has a high catabolic capacity and within milliseconds can increase its metabolic rate 1000-fold from 0.2 to 200 kJ/min approximately. This very high rate of energy expenditure is only possible for up to 10 seconds at the most, since there is an inverse relation between catabolic rate and duration of activity (Fig. 7.1) but, in theory at least, muscle poses a homoeostatic threat. It is not surprising that there are multiple mechanisms for controlling the metabolic activity of muscle cells and also for maintaining whole body homoeostasis during physical activity.

Ordinary exercise such as running, which involves large masses of muscle, creates profound metabolic disturbances; it redistributes blood flow, depletes available energy substrates, increases heat load, and produces large changes in plasma levels of substances such as potassium and lactic acid. A number of adjustments must combine smoothly under neural and hormonal control to

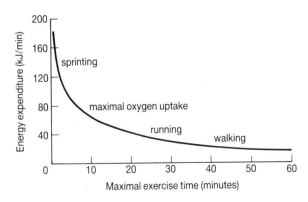

Fig. 7.1 Typical intensity duration curve for dynamic exercise with large muscle mass

allow the large through-put of energy required by vigorous muscular activity, whilst maintaining the internal environment within its normal limits. This is usually successful; exceptions are heat exhaustion or heat stroke which may occur when ambient temperatures are high, water intake is inadequate and exercise is unreasonably prolonged. There is also a rare pathological response to certain anaesthetics in genetically vulnerable individuals in which ATP hydrolysis is uncoupled from muscle contraction and becomes uncontrolled. Heat production is so great that it can lead rapidly to hyperthermia and death. This is a dramatic example of the power of this energy releasing system. This chapter will deal first with energy flows within the muscle cell and then within the whole body. It will be concerned with normal ranges of exercise, referring to the special circumstances of high level athletic performance for illustrative reasons only.

Muscle cells

Functional histology

Three major sub-types of muscle cell (or muscle fibre) are recognized in man, Type I slow oxidative (SO), Type IIb fast glycolytic (FG) and an intermediate Type IIa known as fast oxidative glycolytic (FOG). These three cell types contain different isoenzymes of myosin in their contractile protein, which can be distinguished histologically, and this is associated with varying functional and metabolic characteristics (Table 7.1):

Table 7.1   Variations in muscle cells

Type I (SO)	*Type IIA (FOG)*	*Type IIB (FG)*
Slow	Rate of force development	Fast
Slow	Rate of relaxation	Fast
Low	Rate of stimulation	High
High	Oxidative capacity	Low
High	Capillarity	Low
High	Fatigue resistance	Low
Low	Glycolytic capacity	High
Low	Rate of power output	High
Low	Rate of lactic acid production	High

1. Type I (SO) fibres
   Compared to the others, these contain less myosin ATPase and less sarcoplasmic reticulum with less Ca^{++} release on stimulation. They are slower to develop force and also slower to relax, so they reach a fused tetanic response at a lower frequency of stimulation which is economic for their neural control. They contain higher concentrations of oxidative enzymes, and have an abundant capillary supply which makes them resistant to fatigue. They have smaller motor units and their

motor neurones have a lower firing threshold, so they are the first to be recruited in muscular effort and can easily be sensitively controlled. They are therefore well adapted for the prolonged low energy output and small continuous adjustments required of postural muscles.

2. Type IIb (FG) fibres

These are at the other end of the range in all these respects. In addition they contain higher concentrations of glycolytic enzymes. Consequently they can generate high forces rapidly, but also fatigue rapidly because of their poor oxidative capacity. They require high rates of stimulation and their motor units are large, so control of force output is coarse. They are recruited when relatively large amounts of force or high energy output is required, and so are brought into play only intermittently. They are slightly larger cells and are thought to produce more force/cross-sectional area, either because they contain more contractile protein per unit cross-section or because the myosin type is intrinsically able to generate more force.

3. Type IIb (FOG) fibres

These are intermediate and can adapt, to become more glycolytic or more oxidative according to the demands of customary activity.

These differences in fibre type are reflected to some extent in whole muscles. White muscles contain mainly FG fibres, for example the wing muscles of chickens which are used intermittently. Red muscles, so named because of their vascularity, contain mainly SO fibres, for example, the leg muscles of chickens which must remain active continuously as these birds roost to sleep. Most human muscles are mixed, but soleus and psoas which are postural muscles are predominantly SO, whereas extensor digitorum longus and biceps are predominantly FG. Quadriceps average out at 50 per cent fast and 50 per cent slow but sprinters have a higher and marathon runners a lower proportion of FG fibres. Twin studies have shown that these variations are largely genetically determined. Animal studies have shown that FG fibres can be made slower and more oxidative by stimulating them continuously with a pattern appropriate for SO postural muscle cells, but this happens to a limited extent in man as far as we know.

Metabolic substrates and energy supply

The energy for cross-bridge cycling and generation of force by the actin and myosin complex comes from hydrolysis of ATP. This energy release happens in brief pulses of pico-seconds duration. Turnover of ATP is enormous but stores are small, therefore rapid resynthesis is critical. Phosphocreatine provides this in the short term but it is also limited in amount so breakdown of the large energy stores of glycogen and fat is necessary for activity of more than a few seconds' duration. A summary is given in Fig. 7.2.

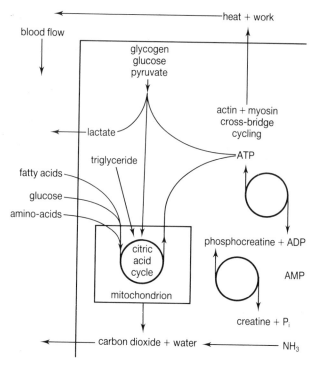

Fig. 7.2 Energy flows in a muscle cell

Glucose

There are glycogen stores in the muscle amounting to about 4.6 MJ which can be metabolized anaerobically as far as pyruvate, yielding 2 moles of ATP per mole of glucose. In the presence of oxygen this enters the citric acid cycle to yield a further 38 moles of ATP per mole of glucose. If there is insufficient oxygen present, 2 moles of pyruvate form one of lactic acid which diffuses out of the muscle cell down its concentration gradient into the interstitial fluid and then into the plasma. Lactate can be taken up and used as a metabolic substrate either locally by other muscle cells if they have oxygen available, or by the liver or the heart. Type I fibres with their greater oxidative capacity probably take up and metabolize lactate released by Type II fibres during moderate exercise. Lactate is also used anabolically in the liver in gluconeogenesis (muscle cells lack the enzymes for this). During moderate exercise when the system is in steady state, rates of lactate production are low and ATP is supplied mainly from the citric acid cycle. This requires transport of glucose or 2-carbon acetyl fragments across the mitochondrial membrane and the diffusion of ATP out in exchange. The glycogen stores will gradually run down despite contributions from fat. Meanwhile plasma glucose is maintained from the much larger stores in the liver. There is thus a possible exchange of lactate for glucose between the liver and the muscle, this is the Cori cycle (Fig. 7.3).

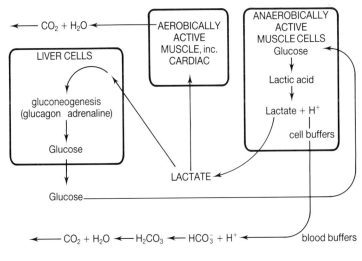

Fig. 7.3 Fate of lactic acid produced during anaerobic exercise

Lactic acid

In exhausting exercise the rate of formation of lactic acid exceeds the rate of diffusion so it accumulates in the muscle cells and reduces their pH from 7.0 to 6.4 despite buffering by bicarbonate, phosphate, and proteins. The very low pH may inhibit the flow of energy in various ways, but it is not now thought to be the primary cause of fatigue in high intensity exercise. Evidence for this includes the finding that recovery of peak force after sustained maximal muscle contraction to exhaustion is independent of pH; the force and phosphocreatine recover completely within a few minutes whilst pH is still very low. Moreover, patients with McArdle's disease who are not able to produce lactic acid suffer from fatigue.

Insulin

This is the anabolic hormone necessary for uptake and storage of glucose in liver and muscle in resting conditions after food ingestion. Insulin release is inhibited during exercise and it is likely therefore that the resulting low plasma insulin levels are permissive of catabolic activity in muscle, liver and adipose tissue. This happens for several reasons. Glucose uptake from plasma into liver cells and non-active muscle is reduced, which conserves whole body glucose, protecting this source of energy for the tissues such as the brain which depend essentially upon it. Active muscle is better able to absorb glucose from plasma than resting muscle and so in prolonged exercise it can draw upon an external supply of glucose as well as its internal stores. There will be a slow rate of release of glucose into the plasma from the liver glycogen stores and from liver gluconeogenesis which is stimulated primarily by glucagon and also by adrenaline.

Free fatty acids

The fat stores in the body represent an enormous energy store. An average man, weighing 70 kg, may contain 10 kg of fat (15 per cent). This represents a store of over 300 MJ. There is a small store of triglyceride in the muscle cell but the rest of the fat substrate must diffuse in from the plasma. Catecholamine release and inhibition of insulin favour lipolysis so there is no shortage of non-esterified free fatty acids (NEFA) circulating in the plasma. However only a modest proportion of the energy used by the muscle cells comes from fat. During high intensity exercise of short duration almost none of it comes from fat because the FG fibres are doing most of the work and oxygen supplies are inadequate to meet the needs of the citric acid cycle. The energy comes from glycolysis such that lactic acid accumulates rapidly. Even during moderate prolonged exercise when the muscle is in aerobic balance the proportion of fat to glucose used never reaches more than 50 per cent and may be as little as 30 per cent. This is evident from RQ measurements (see Glossary, p. 110). It seems that even in the presence of oxygen the citric acid cycle cannot continue on 2-carbon fragments from fat perhaps because some of the intermediates in the cycle are derived from glucose and are catabolized from time to time and so need to be replaced. Individuals who are used to prolonged exercise, and women and those who are in negative energy balance are better able to use fat. Clearly the better individuals are at using fat the better they will be as a marathon runner, other things being equal. It is an unexplained paradox that the body can reach exhaustion because glucose is running out when energy stored as fat is still abundant.

Protein

There are considerable shifts of amino acids in and out of muscle cells during and after exercise. Branched chain amino acids can be used as energy substrates since they can contribute 4-carbon fragments to the citric acid cycle, but their contribution is small in those who are well nourished (see Chapter 2). During prolonged exercise about 10 per cent of the energy comes from this source.

Cortisol and growth hormone

These are released during prolonged or strenuous exercise and favour release of energy substrates (Table A3). In the short term, growth hormone increases lipolysis and it may also have an anabolic role in adults in the long-term response to training.

Muscle cell fatigue

Internal energy stores will support high rates of work for about 30 seconds, but this leads to decrease of phosphocreatine (despite the presence of some remaining glycogen), increases of ADP, AMP, P_i and NH_3, a build up of lactic acid inside the cell, and accumulation of potassium ions outside the cell. The muscle has become fatigued.

The accumulation of extracellular potassium is due to its leakage out of the muscle cell down its concentration gradient when the membrane permeability is temporarily increased after each action potential in order to restore the membrane potential. This imbalance will usually be restored by the sodium/potassium pump, but in strenuous exercise the pump cannot keep pace with the rate of loss. There may also be stimulation of a potassium pump by adrenaline. It is thought that high concentrations of potassium in the transverse tubules prevent membrane depolarization from reaching the interior of the cell to trigger release of calcium ions. Force failure occurs whilst the membrane is still capable of conducting muscle action potentials.

The depletion of phosphocreatine runs in close parallel with the loss of force in repeated maximal contractions. As fatigue develops and force can no longer be generated, even by direct electrical stimulation of the muscle, the ATP turnover rate cannot match the energy demand. At this stage phosphocreatine has been used up, resulting in increased ADP which probably inhibits cross-bridge cycling by occupying the ATP sites. This would explain why the cell fatigues without much fall in ATP levels. The ratio of ADP to ATP may be the critical factor. Creatine ingestion is thought to increase short-term energy output and reduce NH_3 production, by improving the rate of rephosphorylation (Fig. 7.2). Creatine kinase controls the rephosphorylation of creatine and the glycolytic pathway is strongly stimulated by the immediate breakdown products of ATP (AMP, ADP, P_i).

Lower rates of work allow a progressively greater share of the energy expenditure to come from oxidation of glucose and fat. If a balance can be struck between the rate of delivery of oxygen and the energy output then the muscle cell activity can continue for many hours. The end products are water, carbon dioxide (which is eliminated in exchange for oxygen) and heat. There may be small amounts of lactate produced, depending on the intensity of the exercise, but this will not accumulate. Thermoregulatory mechanisms are usually adequate (see below).

Muscle cell response to increased use

Chronic overload, meaning extra use of a muscle, often called training, provides a regular anabolic stimulus which induces RNA. It is not clear exactly what the trigger is. Rest periods between exercise bouts are important for these anabolic processes to happen. The effects are, on the whole local, specific to the muscles used and the type of exercise. Muscle cells respond to extra use by increasing the concentrations of contractile protein and cytosolic glycolytic enzymes in response to increased high intensity exercise (FG), or by increasing oxidative enzymes, mitochondrial density and capillary supply in response to increased prolonged moderate exercise (SO). The muscle cell–capillary diffusing distance shortens with endurance exercise because of proliferation of the capillary network. It is obvious from the differences in recruitment pattern of the fibre types that the kind of exercise needs to be specific. The intermediate fibres will respond accordingly to the kind of exercise, becoming

Table 7.2 24-hour energy expenditure for a 70 kg person: contributions to an average day

	kJ/min	Hours	MJ
Lying down	4.5	9	2.43
Sitting	6.0	6	2.16
Pottering	8.0	7.5	3.60
Walking	16.0	2	1.92
Running	60.0	0.5	1.80
Total			11.91

These rates for various tasks cost more in large individuals and less in small but if they were expressed per kg body mass they would vary little with sex or age in adults. However, the composition of the body changes with sex and age. Women carry more fat at any age and the proportion of fat rises with age in both men and women in affluent countries. Fat is less metabolically active so as lean mass falls with age there is a slight drop in total metabolic rate. In addition all figures quoted as expenditures for tasks will depend upon how enthusiastically they are pursued. Running speeds and rates of work vary enormously. The example is given to show the way different physical activities contribute to total energy expenditure. Low cost prolonged activities make the biggest contribution and high energy activities make rather little because they are brief.

more oxidative in response to endurance exercise and more glycolytic in response to high intensity intermittent sprint training. It is not possible to train a muscle in both directions.

Glycogen loading

Supercompensation of glycogen stores can happen if the glycogen stores are first depleted (over 4 days) using a combination of endurance exercise with a low carbohydrate and high fat diet and then replenished (over 3 days) with very high carbohydrate intake and minimal exercise. This manoeuvre can sometimes double glycogen stores on a temporary basis which will greatly enhance a marathon performance. However, not all individuals respond and the diet is tedious.

Whole body responses

Exercise includes a wide range of activities which have different effects on the body. It includes sprinting for the bus, hill walking, the intermittent activity of field sports, weight training, gymnastics or yoga. It is therefore necessary to specify the kind of exercise under discussion not only in terms of its intensity and duration, but also how much muscle is active and whether the work is steady and rhythmic as in running, intermittent as in squash, or static as in holding up a shelf. Short-term energy output in static work and sprinting will be mentioned later but emphasis will be on the steady rhythmic exercise which can be continued for minutes or hours, often called endurance exercise and which confers stamina. The energy costs of various activities of this kind are given in Table 7.2. The negative relation between the duration and intensity of any kind of dynamic exercise is illustrated in Fig. 7.1

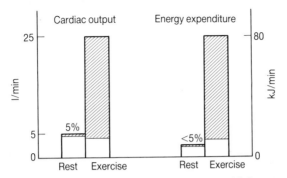

Hatched areas for muscle share; note large increase with exercise especially for energy expenditure (20% of this from anaerobic sources). Open area for the rest of the body, note small fall with exercise in blood flow to the rest of the body along with a small rise in energy expenditure (some of this may be anaerobic).

Fig. 7.4 Changes after 6 min of maximal steady state dynamic exercise such as running i.e. at maximal oxygen uptake

Response to endurance exercise

The response to endurance exercise requires a smoothly coordinated adjustment in many body systems in order to supply the working muscles with an increase of up to 10-fold in their energy consumption (Fig. 7.4). Exercise with the large muscle mass of the legs and trunk used in activities like running, walking, swimming, or cycling will be considered since the amount of muscle in the arms is too small to present a challenge to the homoeostatic mechanisms of whole body. The muscle fibres recruited will be Type I (SO) with the addition of Type II (FOG and FG) depending on the exercise intensity. The latter may produce some lactic acid and whether this accumulates or not depends upon its rate of production which depends in turn on the intensity of the exercise and also its rate of uptake into other tissues.

Redistribution of blood flow and control of blood pressure

A resting muscle requires only a small blood flow since its resting metabolic rate is low. At rest muscle tissue receives about 5 per cent of the cardiac output. When muscle becomes active a number of mechanisms interact to increase muscle blood flow, until at maximal levels of steady exercise, such as running for 6 minutes, the muscle blood flow has increased 20-fold and is taking 80 per cent of the cardiac output (Fig. 7.4). These adjustments take several minutes.

Autoregulation in the muscle will produce local vasodilatation soon after the onset of exercise. This is thought to be mediated by local metabolites from the exercising muscle, however the necessary relaxation of constrictor tone must happen upstream and it happens very rapidly. It is possible that local neuro-humoral reflexes are responsible and that endothelium derived relaxing

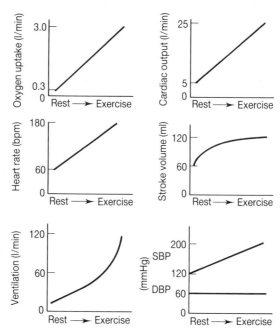

The x-axis represents a graded increase in energy expenditure from rest (6 kJ/min) to vigorous dynamic exercise (80 kJ/min e.g. maximal oxygen uptake).

Fig. 7.5 Energy expenditure and cardio-respiratory response

factor (nitric oxide or a metabolite) may be involved. Whatever the explanation this is a local effect. Since the volume of muscle is large, all the extensor and flexor muscles of the lower half of the body for instance, the vasodilatation of this muscle vasculature would constitute a large decrease in total peripheral resistance if there were no compensatory vasoconstriction elsewhere. However, blood pressure is well maintained because the onset of exercise is accompanied by autonomic changes of central origin, mainly noradrenergic alpha-receptor activity, which selectively vasoconstricts the vasculature in the gut and skin as well as contributing to the increase in cardiac output. There is also a degree of venoconstriction. Since the veins are capacitance vessels a small venoconstriction will increase the venous return to the heart substantially and contribute to the circulating blood volume. This combined with the pumping action of the leg muscles ensures an adequate venous return without which the sympathetic stimulation of the heart could not result in an increased cardiac output. The net effect is an increase in systolic pressure and a maintenance of diastolic pressure amounting to a modest rise in mean blood pressure which preserves blood supply to the enormously dilated muscle capillary network (Fig. 7.5). Adrenaline release contributes to this by increasing heart rate and stroke volume, and may also vasodilate muscle vasculature through its effects on $beta_2$-receptors. The activity of the gut is inhibited and parasympathetic activity is low which can present problems for ingestion of adequate water, salts and glucose in prolonged activity like a marathon run.

Oxygen consumption

This is a measure of the overall metabolic rate, provided the body is in steady state. During exercise most of the oxygen is being delivered to the working muscles but some will be used for metabolism of lactate elsewhere and some for the extra work being done by the heart and the respiratory muscles. If muscle cells are to operate using aerobic energy systems without producing significant amounts of lactic acid at a rate which would accumulate, then the oxygen uptake must match the increased energy expenditure. (There will be small variations in the oxygen need for a given energy expenditure depending on the proportions of fat and glucose used.)

Table 7.3   Energy equivalents for oxygen according to substrate

RQ	kJ obtained from each litre of oxygen (STPD)
1.00	21.13
0.95	20.82
0.90	20.62
0.85	20.36
0.80	20.10
0.75	19.84
0.70	19.58

Cardiac output rises by much less than the oxygen uptake as the oxygen extraction from capillary blood in the muscle doubles. Muscle cells are able to reduce the intracellular partial pressure of oxygen to very low levels and the diffusing distance between the muscle cells and the capillary is shortened due to vasodilatation and increased blood flow. Venous blood draining from an active muscle has a much lower oxygen tension than mixed venous blood. Local acidity, heat and raised carbon dioxide levels affect oxy-haemoglobin, shifting its dissociation curve to the right, which favours oxygen uptake at the muscle cell.

Ventilation increases to maintain the partial pressure of oxygen in the alveoli of the lung whilst much higher volumes of oxygen diffuse across to resaturate the arterial blood to its usual 98 per cent. During moderate exercise these increases match the increase in metabolic rate, but in strenuous exercise there is hyper-ventilation which removes extra carbon dioxide in order to control the acidity produced by lactic acid (Figs. 7.3 and 7.5).

Centres in the medulla function as final common pathways for neural control of the circulatory and ventilatory systems. Integration of many afferent signals with central command from higher levels in the brain occur here. The main afferent signals come from the working muscles triggered by mechanical stimuli and metabolic end products of exercise, including potassium ions.

Maximal oxygen uptake has been widely used in exercise physiology to describe the total capability of the delivery system involving lungs, heart,

Table 7.4 Vigorous endurance exercise which would elicit maximal oxygen uptake

	Rest	Running	Increase
Energy expenditure (kJ)	6.0	72	12×
Oxygen uptake (l/min)*	0.3	3.5	12×
Cardiac output (l/min)*	5	25‡	5×
Heart rate (bpm)	60	180†	3×
Stroke volume (ml)	70	120	<2×
Blood pressure (mm Hg)†			
systolic	120	200	<2×
diastolic	60	60	0
Ventilation (l/min)*	7	120	>12×‡

Variations *with skeletal size, † with age, ‡ with endurance training (see also Table 7.4)

These are typical rounded figures for a young person of average size who is used to exercise. Rest means sitting quietly and exercise means running continuously at a rate which can be continued for 6 minutes (to allow the responses to rise to their plateau). Over the lower ranges of steady exercise, between rest and maximal oxygen uptake, most of these responses will be linearly related to energy expenditure, (oxygen uptake, cardiac output, heart rate and blood pressure). Diastolic pressure may drop very slightly during moderate exercise. Stroke volume rises from 70 to 100 ml in gentle exercise with only a small further increase as exercise becomes strenuous. Ventilation rises linearly until energy expenditure is at about 50 per cent of maximal oxygen uptake; after this plasma lactic acid levels rise rapidly and so does ventilation (the anaerobic threshold has been reached). See also Fig. 7.5.

circulation and muscle. This is achieved in dynamic exercise with large muscle groups such as running. The limits lie in the cardiac output and possibly in constraints on it provided by the baroreceptor system unless the skeletal muscles are very underused. It has been shown in contrived experiments that maximal oxygen uptake during work performed with two legs is not twice the maximal oxygen uptake found when working with one leg, as might be expected, but much less. This shows that the maximal rate at which the leg muscles can take up and use oxygen greatly exceeds the rate at which it is normally delivered when blood flow has to be shared between both working legs in normal modes of activity. The limits must therefore be in the blood flow to the leg. Maximal oxygen uptake is only reached during vigorous exercise when Type II (FG) fibres have also been recruited and about 20 per cent of the energy is coming from anaerobic sources, i.e. there is an excess of energy output over oxygen supply. This situation is not a true steady state and can only continue for 5 or 6 minutes before fatigue sets in for the usual reasons. A numerical summary is given in Table 7.4.

Central effects of training

Maximal cardiac output increases because maximal stroke volume increases but there is no change in maximal heart rate or ventilation. The stroke volume goes up partly because improved cardiac contractility allows more complete emptying, there may be a small increase in plasma volume and a slight increase in cardiac dimensions. Prolonged intensive endurance training leads to increases of about 10 per cent in the internal dimensions of the heart, wall thickness and weight of heart muscle. More modest levels of training may induce smaller

Table 7.5 Variations in response to exercise (see also Table 7.3)

	Age	Size	Training
Maximal level – 6 minutes of running			
Maximal oxygen uptake	Down	Up	Up
Cardiac output	Down	Up	Up
Stroke volume	—	Up	Up
Heart rate	Down	—	—
Ventilation	Down	Up	—
Blood pressure	Varies	—	—
Submaximal level – walking briskly up a 5% gradient			
Cardiac output	—	—	—
Stroke volume	—	Up	Up
Heart rate	—	Down	Down
Ventilation	—	Down	—
Blood pressure	—	Down	Down

improvements which are functionally relevant, but below the limits of detection by echocardiographic techniques. Large increases in cardiac size would in theory be counter-productive and in practice are found to be pathological. For instance moderately increased internal dimensions require considerably increased wall tension to achieve the same internal pressure, because the wall tension increases as the square of the internal dimensions. Increases in wall thickness are limited by diastolic perfusion time. If the wall is too thick the cardiac capillary flow does not have time to reach the deepest layers so the thickened ventricular muscle wall of a hypertensive patient often causes ischaemic pain. These variations are summarized in Table 7.5.

During sub-maximal exercise, i.e. performing a given task which has the same energy cost before and after training, heart rate decreases for the same reasons. Improvements in the muscle and muscle cells will have secondary effects on the cardiorespiratory system. There is reduced peripheral drive if the muscle is better able to take up and use oxygen and central command will decrease if fewer motor units are needed to do the same work because of increases in muscle strength. There is no intrinsic change in the efficiency of energy transformations in the muscle cells. There may be an apparent change in efficiency because the same task is now performed with more skill and less wasted external energy (Table 7.5).

In high intensity dynamic activity

In such a situation (e.g. sprinting) the anaerobic capacity determines maximal energy expenditure. This depends on how much muscle is being used, on the proportion of Type II fibres and the concentration of glycolytic enzymes within them. Fatigue in high intensity activity is due to an inadequate rate of ATP replenishment, and an associated rising ADP/ATP ratio which stops further cross-bridge cycling (see Muscle cell fatigue). Recovery is rapid when exercise stops. Intermittent exercise allows periods of intense anaerobic exercise interspersed with brief periods of less intense aerobic exercise during which the oxygen debt which has been accumulated is paid back, lactate is removed and the oxygen stores replenished. This mode of exercising is typical of many sports, and work situations and allows the largest through-put of energy. Within limits, the shorter the duty cycles of rest and exercise the better. Half-minute cycles allow a given mean rate of work to proceed with a much lower heart rate and lower lactate levels than 3-minute cycles.

Static work

This is different from all other kinds of exercise. The muscle is contracted isometrically, there is no perceptible movement, and if the contraction is above 25–30 per cent of the muscle's own maximum strength and is maintained, the muscle force can restrict its own blood supply. This leads to rapid local fatigue (see above) and pain so severe that static contractions last a few minutes at the most. Weaker individuals may do better and training which improves strength will reduce the duration of maintained contraction because the muscle now blocks its own blood flow even more effectively. Heart rate and mean blood pressure rise continually whilst the contraction is maintained and small muscles can elicit sharp responses. This can be viewed as a fruitless attempt to provide perfusion. It is a reflex response initiated from the ischaemic muscle probably by increased interstitial potassium stimulating free nerve endings in muscle tissue. The afferents are Group C fibres which influence the medullary control centres.

Postural muscles are in a more or less permanent state of contraction; however, because they are operating at a low proportion of their maximal capability (less than 20 per cent) their blood supply is adequate and they remain in aerobic balance.

Control of heat loads

The efficiency of energy conversion from substrate to external work in muscular exercise is about 20 per cent, which means that 80 per cent of the energy is released as heat. This can cause problems during prolonged vigorous exercise in warm climatic conditions. Heat must be distributed by the circulation from its source and lost to the environment through the skin and lungs, and heat loss must equal heat production to keep the core of the body within very narrow limits, usually between 36° and 37°C. Resting metabolic rate represents continuous heat production which is useful for maintaining core temperature in a cold environment but becomes a heat load in a warm environment. Exercise can increase this load 10-fold over short time periods and significantly increase the heat content of the body. Core temperature is allowed to rise in prolonged exercise but in a controlled manner and in proportion to the intensity of the exercise. The rectal temperature of a marathon runner may reach 41°C; however, his aural or oesophageal temperature may not be so elevated since much of the abdominal heat gain is due to heated blood coming from the active lower body musculature.

Control of body temperature

This is mainly neural. The skin has abundant temperature sensitive nerve endings, covering varying ranges of temperature, which relay to the spinal cord to produce local vasodilatation and to the hypothalamus to contribute to central integration. They are rapidly adapting, like most sensory neurones, and so sense changes rather than steady state. They are therefore not useful for primary control but necessary as modulators of central mechanisms. Their ability to initiate reflex vasodilatation at spinal level is a local protection against excessive cold but it is subservient to central control. The sensation of thermal comfort or otherwise is important as it leads to behavioural modification. We create a micro-climate inside our clothes and our buildings. Thermal comfort depends on an ambient temperature of about 25°C with air velocity low (0.2/m.s) and humidity 30–75 per cent with even heat distribution in the room.

Central control is provided by groups of thermosensitive neurones in the hypothalamus which have a set point temperature. This can be influenced by input from the periphery. Temperature signals from many parts of the body are integrated in the hypothalamus, these signals came from the spinal cord and arterial tree, as well as the skin. The efferent pathways are through autonomic control of skin vasoconstrictor tone (sympathetic noradrenergic), which continuously adjusts the core–skin gradient (0–20°C), and sweat rate (sympathetic cholinergic).

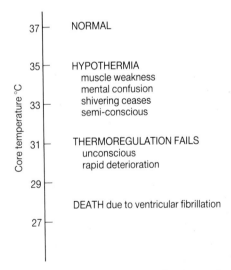

Fig. 7.6 Hypothermia defined as core temp < 35°C

Heat loss

Heat loss can occur through conduction, convection, radiation or evaporation depending on local conditions. Air movement increases convection and so aids heat loss. Sweating is a very effective mechanism for heat loss, provided the humidity is low enough to allow the water to evaporate from the skin surface. Sweat which is standing as visible drops on the skin is not removing heat from the body. The latent heat of evaporation of the sweat can dissipate heat from the body even in the face of high ambient temperatures. However, the increased skin blood flow puts further demands on the cardiac output for a share of the blood flow to the skin. Sweat rates can be as high as two litres (equivalent to 5 MJ of heat loss) per hour in the short term or one litre per hour for many hours. These losses are large compared to a total blood volume of 6 litres, so there will be marked ADH release and oliguria. There is also increased water loss from the lungs due to increased ventilation and a shift of water from plasma into the muscle interstitial fluid. This occurs because of increased concentrations of metabolites produced by the working muscle cells and an adrenaline-mediated increase in capillary permeability which allows albumin to escape. Both exercise capacity and heat tolerance will be reduced if central blood volume falls. Blood pressure must be maintained so fluid and salt replacement are critical. The success of this homoeostasis depends crucially on adequate hydration and maintenance of blood volume.

Acclimatization to heat occurs after 2–3 weeks of exposure to hot environments. Sweat rate increases (2-fold), sweating begins earlier, i.e. at a lower threshold core temperature, blood volume increases, salt is conserved (loss in sweat and urine reduced). Tolerance for exercise is therefore greatly improved.

Heat exhaustion occurs when there is insufficient blood volume to support adequate blood flow for both skin and muscle. Circulatory control becomes precarious, blood pressure falls so the skin vessels vasoconstrict and core temperature rises. The victim needs to rest in a supine position with elevated legs. Fluid replacement and external cooling must be administered with as little delay as possible. If this happens recovery is usually complete.

Heat stroke is a much more serious version of heat exhaustion in which loss of thermoregulatory control leads to rapid rise in core temperature, loss of full consciousness and a rising metabolic rate due to the increased core temperature. A positive feedback has developed which will be rapidly fatal if external intervention cannot reduce the core temperature. Vigorous cooling with ice packs, and fluid replacement has a chance, but hospitalization is required for adjustment of fluid, and acid–base balance and dialysis may be needed. The outcome depends on speed and efficacy of treatment, there may be full recovery or widespread (often irreversible) damage to neurones, blood vessels, and the kidney.

Fever

Hyperthermia occurs in pathological states produced by toxins from bacteria and viruses which increase prostaglandin levels in the hypothalamus and so perturb the temperature regulating control centres. Conscious sensation is also affected, so the patient feels cold, and may even shiver despite raised core temperature and warm skin. Treatment with drugs such as aspirin returns the controls to normal by inhibiting prostaglandin synthesis.

Heat conservation

In *cold conditions* heat loss is decreased by vasoconstricting the skin, the temperature of peripheral tissues (hands and feet) is allowed to drop well below core temperature, heat is conserved by the counter-current heat exchange between the arteries and veins which run to the periphery together, and if core temperature drops below normal there is increased heat production by shivering. This only happens if the skin is cold; input from cold receptors in skin is necessary to facilitate the hypothalamic neurones which initiate shivering. Shivering consists of synchronous activity of small groups of motor neurones without gross movements; this can treble the metabolic rate. There is no good evidence that true cold acclimatization occurs in man.

Slow cooling typically happens in hill-walkers when the weather deteriorates, clothing is inadequate, and exercise capability has been over-estimated. Heat loss begins to exceed heat production. Muscle weakness and mental confusion develop slowly and progressively, which impairs behavioural response. Skin temperature receptors have adapted so there is no cold signal to the hypothalamic control centres and so no shivering (Fig. 7.6). The best advice is to ensure insulation against cold and wind chill, protect against hypoglycaemia, and avoid alcohol which impairs gluconeogenesis. Treatment is to prevent further heat loss as far as possible, then warm slowly (in bed in a warm room). A sudden influx of cold, acidic, hyperkalaemic blood from the periphery may cause ventricular fibrillation so ECG monitoring is desirable. Premature warming of cold extremities before their blood supply has returned causes severe ischaemia because the local metabolic rate goes up whilst the tissue is still deprived of oxygen and glucose. Survival of tissues depends on keeping metabolic rate in balance with metabolic supply of oxygen and substrates.

Rapid cooling typically happens with unexpected immersion in cold water (boating accidents or shipwreck). Survival time depends on water temperature and body insulation (fat + clothing) (Table 7.6). Water conducts heat much more rapidly than air. The best advice is not to swim as this increases loss through convection. The small thin people should be saved first, i.e. children and thin young men. Women, especially the middle-aged, will survive for longer because they have more subcutaneous fat. Treatment is to warm relatively

Table 7.6 Survival time on immersion in water

Sea temperature (°C)	Survival time (min)	
	Naked	Clothed
5	10–15	20–60
15	20–60	5 hours

rapidly with inhalation of warmed air; there is a risk of ventricular fibrillation just as for slow cooling. There have been anecdotal accounts of complete recovery after many hours of apparent death due to hypothermia. The crucial consideration is the match between the metabolic rate of the tissue, especially neural tissue, and its supply of oxygen and nutrients. Death of tissues occurs primarily because of ischaemia following cardiac arrest. This is exemplified by the use of controlled reversible hypothermia in open heart surgery. The circulation is artificially cooled to reduce the metabolic rate until the heart stops so that complex intervention is possible.

Vulnerable groups

Babies are vulnerable to cold conditions because they can lose heat rapidly due to their high ratio of surface area to volume and their, as yet, undeveloped ability to shiver. However, they are protected to some extent by specialized brown adipose tissue with a rich vasculature and mitochondria which can become uncoupled. This tissue is sensitive to catecholamines which stimulate, in a controlled manner, uncoupled ATP breakdown which can produce a great deal of heat (c.f. anaesthetically-induced hyperthermia). The adrenaline is released in response to cold conditions (cold skin and/or reduced core temperature). Adults have some brown fat but it is not clear whether they have the ability to use it for survival in cold conditions. Babies also deal with heat less effectively because of immature sweat glands. Old people are more vulnerable in both heat and cold. They are alleged to be less sensitive to both and therefore may not respond behaviourally. They are less active and so produce less heat and they have a lower capacity for sweating.

Hazards and health benefits of exercise

Sustained muscle contraction produces a steep and continuing rise in mean blood pressure. High intensity activity may damage muscles, tendons and ligaments, especially in violent contact sports or eccentric work (running downhill for example). Energy is absorbed in eccentric contractions so the energy expenditure is small and there is no metabolic threat but the muscle forces are high. Prolonged aerobic exercise or repetitive intermittent exercise can lead to over-use injuries such as stress fractures, inflamed tendons or arthritic changes in joints. Prolonged energy expenditure can exhaust glucose stores and lead to collapse due to hypoglycaemia and ionic imbalance. High energy production in hot climatic conditions can lead to heat over-load.

There are also hazards attributable to lack of exercise. Loss of physical capabilities is particularly threatening for older individuals who have smaller safety margins when their physical capabilities are compared to the needs of daily tasks; variety of exercise is needed to preserve function. Without adequate regular endurance exercise there is an increased risk of developing chronic diseases, such as heart disease, diabetes, obesity, and hypertension. Exercises which provide brief, fairly intense bone loading may help to preserve bone density and protect against osteoporosis which afflicts mainly women in later life. In addition, mortality and morbidity in chronic diseases are exacerbated by under-used skeletal muscles which put a greater strain on the cardiorespiratory system.

Glossary

Energy expenditure	= metabolic rate
	= calories 'burned'
	= oxygen consumption (at steady state)
external energy expenditure	= rate of work
	= power output
	= exercise intensity
conversion of units: kcal/min	= 4.2 kJ/min
	= 70 watts
	= 0.21 l/min oxygen consumption (slightly variable depending on substrate)

$$\text{Efficiency of muscular work} = \frac{\text{external energy expenditure (rate of work)}}{\text{total } - \text{ resting energy expenditure}}$$

$$\text{Respiratory quotient} = \frac{\text{carbon dioxide production}}{\text{oxygen consumption}}$$

If assessed at steady state, RQ relates to metabolic substrate (see Table 7.3). In non-steady states or in vigorous exercise, CO_2 loss may exceed production. This occurs during hyperventilation to control pH; the ratio is then called the respiratory exchange ratio (RER) and is no longer a guide to substrate use.

8

Cholesterol metabolism

Atherosclerosis, presenting clinically as coronary heart disease, cerebrovascular disease or peripheral artery disease, is the most frequent cause of death and disability in industrialized countries. A major risk factor in coronary heart disease is hyperlipoproteinaemia and the importance of hypercholesterolaemia as the primary risk factor has been shown in a number of epidemiological studies. The results of many intervention trials at various centres involving thousands of patients have demonstrated that a reduction in serum cholesterol concentration shows a positive correlation with a reduction in the incidence of coronary heart disease. But whilst cholesterol may be seen as an 'enfant terrible' by the popular press it should be remembered that it is an essential component of cellular membranes and the precursor of steroid hormones and bile acids.

Cholesterol transport

Cholesterol is transported primarily as cholesterylester in lipoprotein fractions which differ in their buoyant density and a total serum cholesterol value measures the sum of all four fractions (HDL+LDL+IDL+VLDL). Measurement of HDL-cholesterol can be made after first precipitating apoB-containing lipoproteins (VLDL+IDL+LDL) with polyanions such as dextran sulphate, phosphotungstate or heparin and the difference between this value and the total cholesterol represents the VLDL + IDL + LDL cholesterol. An approximate value for LDL-cholesterol can be calculated by inserting the HDL and total cholesterol data in the Friedwald formula

$$\text{LDL-C} = \text{Total-C} - \left[\frac{\text{TAG}}{2.2} + \text{HDL-C} \right]$$

which holds true for serum triacylglycerol (TAG) values below 4.6 mM. For most individuals a single total cholesterol measurement is made but in patients with hypercholesterolaemia, HDL- and LDL-cholesterol measurement may be of value in management. As for what should be the optimal blood cholesterol concentration there is something of a disparity between what is desirable and what is achievable, but the NIH Consensus Development Panel and the study group of the European Atherosclerosis Society suggest that 'it is a goal to encourage reduction of blood cholesterol to approximately 180 mg/dl (4.7 mM) for adults under the age of 30 years and to approximately 200 mg/dl (5.2 mM) for individuals aged 30 or older'. The rationale for using various drugs to achieve such values may be understood from a knowledge of processes which contribute to the homoeostatic concentration of cholesterol in the blood.

Whole body cholesterol homoeostasis

The homoeostatic concentration of cholesterol in the plasma, carried by the lipoproteins represents a balance between input from the diet and endogenous synthesis, primarily by the liver and the intestine, and output in the bile as free cholesterol and bile acids (Fig. 8.1). The standardized 70 kg man contains about 60 g of cholesterol of which about two-thirds is present in a stable pool in skin, adipose tissue and muscle. The other one-third is in a more mobile pool circulating in the plasma through the liver. An 'average' diet contributes about 0.5 g cholesterol daily and endogenous synthesis a further 1 g. Since the daily metabolic requirement of cholesterol is around 350 mg the balance has to be excreted via the bile into the faeces or stored in tissues. All nucleated cells have the full complement of enzymes required for cholesterol synthesis and thus there is an excessive synthetic capacity in the body. This endogenous synthesis must be strictly regulated to maintain cholesterol homoeostasis and avoid cholesterol deposition.

The cholesterol available for absorption from the gastrointestinal tract is derived from biliary secretions and desquamated epithelial cells as well as from the diet. Cholesterylesters in the GI tract are hydrolysed by a pancreatic cholesterylesterase and the free cholesterol produced partitions into the mixed micelles of lipids (monoglycerides, lysophospholipids and bile salts) from which absorption, mainly in the jejunum, takes place. A deficiency in bile acid

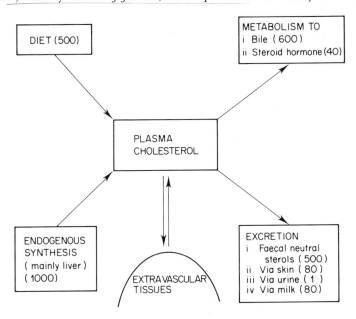

Fig. 8.1 Whole body cholesterol homoeostasis. Figures in parentheses indicate approximate daily throughput in milligrams

secretion leads to malabsorption of cholesterol. In man a high cholesterol intake may not necessarily lead to an increase in plasma cholesterol since the body adapts to changes in dietary cholesterol content. On a low cholesterol intake (400–500 mg/day) about 50 per cent is absorbed while on a high intake (1200–1500 mg/day) only about 30 per cent is absorbed. To offset this increased input there is also an enhancement of neutral sterol excretion in the faeces and decreased endogenous cholesterol synthesis, particularly in the liver. Once inside the enterocyte free cholesterol is re-esterified and secreted as a component of the chylomicron, the metabolism of which is described later.

Metabolism and excretion of cholesterol

The major routes of cholesterol loss are shown in Fig. 8.1. Conversion to the bile acids and conjugation with glycine or taurine in the liver represents the major loss. This process involves the loss of a 3-carbon fragment as propionyl-CoA (Fig. 8.2). However, only about 10 per cent of the bile acid pool is lost each day because the bile acids undergo enterohepatic circulation, being reabsorbed in the distal ileum and cycling about six times a day. Apart from their essential role in micelle formation and lipid absorption in the GI tract, bile salts serve as detergents to solubilize free cholesterol excreted into the bile by the liver. Cholesterol is also the precursor for steroid hormone synthesis in the adrenal cortex and sex glands (Fig. 8.2; as described in Chapter 1) and also for vitamin D.

Detoxication products of steroid metabolism are excreted in the urine, whilst direct loss of cholesterol from biliary secretions, desquamated epithelial cells and non-absorbed dietary cholesterol occurs in the faeces. The total loss of sterol, as bile salts and cholesterol, is between 1.0–1.5 g per day. Other minor losses arise from flaked-off upper layers of stratum corneum and, in lactating mothers, as part of the lipid fraction of milk.

Regulation of cholesterol synthesis

All nucleated cells have the ability to synthesize cholesterol although the intestine and particularly the liver are the major cholesterol-synthesizing tissues. Cholesterol is synthesized from acetyl-CoA via a sequence of 26 steps with the major regulatory step at the site of mevalonate production, 3-hydroxy-3-methylglutarylcoenzymeA reductase (HMGCoAR). Mevalonate

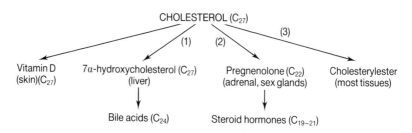

Fig. 8.2 Major routes of cholesterol metabolism
(1) Cholesterol 7α-hydroxylase (2) Desmolase (3) Acylcoenzyme A: cholesterolacyl transferase (ACAT)

is the precursor for a number of other products (Fig. 8.3) and its production is subject to a variety of controls, both acute and chronic, to allow sufficient mevalonate for isoprenoid synthesis without the overproduction of cholesterol. Indeed, the enzymes of the non-sterol pathways have a higher affinity than the sterol pathway for mevalonate-derived substrates such that when mevalonate is limiting it is shunted into the non-sterol pathways.

Since most cells can acquire cholesterol exogenously via receptor-mediated endocytosis of LDL (see below and Fig. 8.7), cellular cholesterol homoeostasis must be achieved by feedback regulation of HMGCoAR, its preceding enzyme HMGCoA synthase and LDL receptors. Thus when LDL supplies cholesterol to the cell the activities of HMGCoA synthase and HMGCoAR are greatly reduced such that sufficient mevalonate is made to satisfy only the synthesis of non-sterol metabolites.

HMGCoAR is an enzyme of the smooth endoplasmic reticulum (SER) where it exists as a dimer of two 97 kDa subunits. It is one of the most highly regulated enzymes, being subject to control both at the level of transcription and post-transcriptionally. These controls which may be endogenous or exogenous can alter the activity of the enzyme and its amount in the cell. Acute control of the enzyme may be brought about by changes in the fluidity of the SER membrane due to cholesterol loading or by a hormone-induced

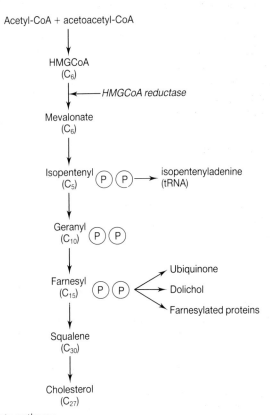

Fig. 8.3 The mevalonate pathway

phosphorylation–dephosphorylation cycle (Fig. 8.4). Phosphorylation of the cAMP-dependent reductase kinase is promoted by glucagon and results in rapid degradation of the enzyme and decreased enzyme mass. Insulin has the opposite effect. The activity of the reductase kinase is also subject to a similar phosphorylation–dephosphorylation control by a reductase kinase kinase.

Sterol regulation of HMGCoAR appears to be at the level of transcription in a manner similar to that of steroid hormones described in Chapter 1. The HMGCoAR gene contains a short sequence, the sterol regulatory element (SRE), in the 5′ flanking region which renders the gene sensitive to the presence of sterols. Thus in the presence of sterols, transcription of the gene is actively repressed. Similar regulatory sequences exist in the 5′ flanking regions of both the LDL receptor and HMGCoA synthase genes. In these two cases, however, transcription is enhanced in the absence, but not in the presence, of sterols. Although not yet described, it is possible that a sterol or oxy-sterol might bind to a DNA-binding protein in the cytosol and promote its translocation to the nucleus and act as a regulator of the sterol regulatory elements. Further control at the level of translation of HMGCoAR messenger RNA is beyond the scope of the current text.

Gallstones

Gallstone formation in the gallbladder is a common disease in western society. It is estimated that between 16 and 20 million Americans have gallstones and in Britain gallstones are found in 10 per cent of all necropsies. Although some (25 per cent) of the stones are pigmented precipitates of calcium salts, greater than 75 per cent are predominantly crystalline cholesterol monohydrate.

The bile is a <u>major excretory route for cholesterol</u> and sterol is maintained

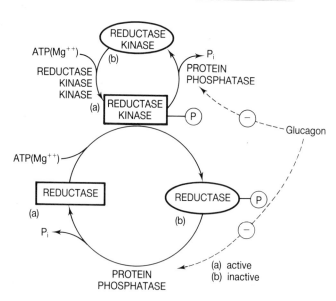

Fig. 8.4 Bicyclic kinase/phosphatase system controlling HMGCoA reductase

in solution by the formation of mixed micelles of lecithin and bile acids. Supersaturation of bile with respect to cholesterol may occur as a consequence of situations which alter the delicate balance of the three lipid classes in bile. For example, increased biliary cholesterol secretion due to increased hepatic cholesterol synthesis or a reduction in the bile acid pool size due to faecal loss or decreased synthesis increase the lithogenicity of bile. In both these instances the liver is at fault and increased HMGCoAR and decreased cholesterol 7α-hydroxylase activities, the rate limiting steps of cholesterol and bile acid synthesis respectively, have been found in patients with cholesterol gallstones. Supersaturation of bile with respect to homoeostasis precedes and predisposes to the formation of cholesterol stones. Increased saturation and a high incidence of gallstone disease is associated with obesity, use of contraceptive steroids and drugs such as clofibrate. The classical at risk group fits the 'six F nemonic' – fair, female, fat, flatulent, fertile and forty.

Precipitation of cholesterol occurs particularly on concentration of bile in the gallbladder. While stones sometimes remain 'silent' and asymptomatic they may obstruct the cystic duct causing cholecystitis and produce biliary cholic, fever and jaundice.

At present cholecystectomy is the usual treatment for gallstones both pigmented and radiolucent (cholesterol) and it has been estimated that more than 400 000 cholecystectomies are performed in the USA each year. However, non-invasive treatments aimed at dissolving cholesterol gallstones by desaturating bile have received much attention. Although *de novo* synthesis of cholesterol in the liver accounts for less than one-third of the biliary cholesterol output, inhibition of this synthesis by oral administration of the primary or secondary bile acids, chenodeoxycholic acid or ursodeoxycholic acid (chenotherapy) in combination with extra-corporeal shock wave lithotripsy, has achieved some success in dissolution of cholesterol stones. In doses which do not contribute significantly to the total bile acid pool the exogenous bile acids appear to desaturate bile by inhibiting hepatic synthesis and secretion of cholesterol. Gallstone patients treated with chenodeoxycholic acid for 6 months had lower hepatic HMGCoAR activities than untreated patients. However, only about 30 per cent of patients with gall bladder disease are suitable for lithotripsy and the treatment is very expensive. A major problem with such chenotherapy is what happens when the drug is discontinued. Dissolution requires prolonged therapy and in many cases on discontinuation the bile returns to its supersaturated state with the recurrence of gallstones.

Lipoproteins

Since lipids by their very nature are hydrophobic, an efficient means of transport of both exogenously- and endogenously-derived lipid through the aqueous environment of the circulation is required. In addition a mechanism for targetting lipids to specific tissues must exist. Lipoproteins provide a vehicle both for transport and for recognition by specific receptors on tissues. In general lipoproteins are spherical in shape, consisting of an oily lipophilic core of cholesterylester and varying amounts of triglyceride surrounded by a monolayer of phospholipids containing proteins (apoproteins) and free cholesterol. They

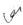

Table 8.1   Major lipoproteins of human plasma

	Chylomicrons	VLDL	IDL	LDL	HDL
Density (g/ml)	<1.000	<1.006	1.006–1.019	1.019–1.063	1.063–1.21
Diameter (nm)	80–100	30–80	25–30	20–25	8–13
Electrophoretic mobility	Uncharged	Pre-β	β	β	α
Major components (%)					
TAG	90–95	50–65	25–40	4–6	7
CE	2–4	8–14	20–35	35–45	10–20
C	1	4–7	7–11	6–15	5
PL	2–6	12–16	16–24	22–26	25
Protein	1–2	5–10	12–16	22–26	45
Major apoproteins (% total protein)	A-I(31) C(32)E(10) B-48(5–8)	C(40–50) B-100(30–40) E(10–15)	B-100(60–80) C(10–20) E(10–15)	B-100(>95) (C<1)E(<1)	A-I(65) A-II(10–23) C(5–15) E(1–3)

are classified into four major groups: chylomicrons (CM); very low density lipoproteins (VLDL); intermediate density lipoproteins (IDL); low density lipoproteins (LDL); and high density lipoproteins (HDL), on the basis of their density which reflects the proportion of lipid in the core and apoprotein content (Table 8.1). This difference in density is used in their isolation by sequential flotation in media of increasing density. A varying apoprotein composition also gives the lipoproteins different charges and thus different electrophoretic mobilites (α-HDL, preβ-VLDL and β-LDL) which may be of diagnostic value in qualitative analysis of lipoproteins in patients with defects in lipoprotein metabolism. The properties of the major apoproteins are shown in Table 8.2. It should be remembered however that a classification into four discrete major subgroups is something of an over-simplification and that lipoproteins are distributed along a density continuum from a density of 1.00 g/ml (chylomicrons) to 1.2 g/ml (high density lipoproteins). Also, lipoproteins are highly dynamic structures whose particle size and composition are undergoing continual change with both lipid and protein moving within and between lipoprotein classes. In describing the metabolism of the lipoproteins the following abbreviations will be used:

1. LPL; lipoprotein lipase, an extracellular enzyme present on the surface of the capillary endothelium which hydrolyses triglyceride to free fatty acids and glycerol. It is synthesized and secreted by muscle and adipose cells and is released from its anchor site by heparin.
2. LCAT; lecithin-cholesterol acyltransferase (68 kDa), an enzyme secreted by the liver which catalyses the formation of cholesterylester from free cholesterol and phosphatidylcholine (lecithin) in HDL. It is activated by apoprotein A-I.
3. CETP; cholesterylester transfer protein (74 kDa), synthesized mainly by the liver, and mediates the transfer of cholesterylester between lipoprotein species, particularly from HDL to remnant particles formed from metabolism of VLDL and chylomicrons.
4. ACAT; acylcoenzyme-A: cholesterol acyltransferase is an enzyme of the endoplasmic reticulum which catalyses the intracellular synthesis of cholesterylester from free cholesterol and acylcoenzyme-A.

Table 8.2 Some properties of the major apoproteins

Apoprotein	Relative mol. wt. (kDa)	Major location	Function
A-I	28 000	HDL, CM	Binding to AI (HDL) receptor. Activator of LCAT.
A-II	17 000		
B-100	512 000	LDL, IDL, VLDL	Binding to LDL (apoB-100) receptor.
B-48	245 000	CM	Assembly of chylomicrons.
C-II	9000	CM, VLDL, IDL, HDL	Binding to and activation of LPL.
E	34 000		Binding to apoE receptor; inhibitor of LPL.

5. CEH; cholesterylester hydrolase, an enzyme which hydrolyses stored cholesterylester to free cholesterol and fatty acid. There are at least two species; an acidic lysosomal enzyme and an enzyme which is active at neutral pH.

Triglyceride-rich lipoproteins

The two largest and least dense lipoproteins are responsible respectively for the transport of diet-derived and endogenously synthesized triglyceride.

Chylomicrons

Chylomicrons (CM) which contain greater than 90 per cent triglyceride by weight are synthesized in the intestine following a meal and the CM concentration reflects the fat content of the meal. Monoacylglycerol and free fatty acids produced by hydrolysis of dietary triglycerides in the lumen of the small intestine are absorbed across the microvilli membranes and triglycerides of composition similar to dietary triglycerides are synthesized in the enterocyte. Formation of the chylomicron also requires synthesis of cholesterylester and apoproteins, particularly apoB-48. Failure to synthesize either of these components will result in non-assembly of the chylomicron particle and lipid will be lost as the enterocyte sloughs off, producing an effective fat malabsorption. Thus patients who are unable to synthesize apoprotein B present with fat malabsorption (steatorrhoea) and also fat-soluble vitamin deficiency since vitamins A, D, E and K are incorporated into the chylomicron for transport to the liver. Indeed, it has been suggested that this transport of dietary fat-soluble vitamins to the liver is a primary role of the chylomicron.

Chylomicrons leave the enterocyte via the lymphatic system and enter the circulation through the thoracic duct (Fig. 8.5). Nascent particles contain apoB-48 and apoAI but are deficient in the C apoproteins which are required for interaction with lipoprotein lipase in the capillary beds of extrahepatic tissues such as adipose tissue and muscle. They acquire apo Cs and apoE, during metabolism, from HDL, an example of intraparticle movement of lipoprotein components mentioned earlier. Interaction of the mature chylomicrons with LPL via apoCII results in extracellular hydrolysis of the core triglyceride to free fatty acids and glycerol. The free fatty acids are taken up by the extrahepatic tissue and either stored as triglyceride or metabolized. Resynthesis of triglyceride in such tissues requires the provision of glycerol-3-phosphate from glycolysis. Chylomicrons are produced in the 'just-fed state', being found in the circulation following a meal at a time when blood glucose and hence insulin concentrations are raised. Insulin, which activates LPL, will also promote the uptake of glucose into the tissue and stimulate glycolysis to provide the glycerol-3-phosphate acceptor of fatty acids derived from LPL hydrolysis of CM-triglyceride for intracellular storage of triglyceride.

Approximately 80–90 per cent of CM-triglyceride is hydrolysed by LPL and loss of triglyceride from the core of the chylomicron leads to a change in the shape and reduction in the size of the particle (chylomicron remnant) with concomitant loss of apoproteins C and AI to HDL. As the affinity for LPL decreases the previously latent apoE is expressed on the remnant particle surface to allow it to interact with apoE receptors on hepatocytes and be cleared by the liver. This clearance may involve some further hydrolysis of remnant triglyceride by the hepatic triglyceride lipase (HTGL). ApoE has a region in the middle of its sequence which is rich in basic amino acids which might also allow some interaction with the apoB LDL receptor. However, the apoB-48 of the remnant will not interact with the apoB receptor since although it is the product of the same gene as apoB-100, post-transcriptional tissue-specific editing in the intestine of nucleotide 6457 of apoB mRNA (CAA→UAA) introduces a termination codon in place of glutamine at amino acid 2153 and terminates the intestinal apoB-48 at amino acid 2152 with a C-terminal isoleucine. This product is approximately 48 per cent (i.e. B-48) of the length of the fully translated apoB (B-100). The LDL receptor binding site resides in the C-terminal region of apoB-100, i.e. within the 52 per cent of the sequence missing in apoB-48. Thus apoB-48 is unable to bind to the LDL receptor. Virtually all CMR are removed as particles of density less than 1.019 g/ml and thus apoB-48 is not normally found in the LDL fraction. Furthermore, since CM have a residence time in the circulation of between 5 and 20 minutes the apoB-48 concentration in plasma is very low and represents no more than 0.1 per cent of total apoB.

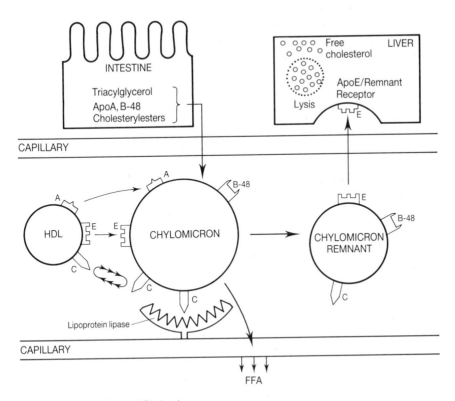

Fig. 8.5 The metabolism of Chylomicrons

Very low density lipoproteins (VLDL)

VLDL are also rich in triglycerides (50–60 per cent by weight) but they are assembled in and secreted by the liver into the space of Disse, entering the circulation via the hepatic vein (Fig. 8.6) The half-life of VLDL is of the order of 30 minutes. The source of fatty acids for VLDL triglycerides is from either adipose tissue or endogenous hepatic synthesis The cholesterylester, phospholipid, free cholesterol and apoprotein (apoB and apoC) content is higher than in CM, although interestingly VLDL appear to contain only a single molecule of apoB-100 and the nascent particle secreted by the liver contains little cholesterylester. Its cholesterylester content increases during metabolism by transfer from HDL, as discussed later. Again all components of the VLDL particle must be synthesized before secretion can occur.

Hydrolysis of VLDL-borne triglyceride occurs, as with CM triglyceride, through the action of the apoCII-activated LPL in the capillaries of peripheral tissues with the concomitant transport of free fatty acids into the tissue. Although the VLDL particles contain apoB-100 this appears to be latent in the nascent and native lipoprotein such that it does not bind to the apoB receptor. As the triglyceride is lost the particle increases in density to intermediate density lipoproteins (IDL) or VLDL remnants (VLDLR) and apoproteins B and E are expressed on the surface. There are two possible fates for the IDL, both of which occur very rapidly such that the plasma concentration of IDL is low in normal individuals. The appearance of apoB and apoE on the particle surface allow it to

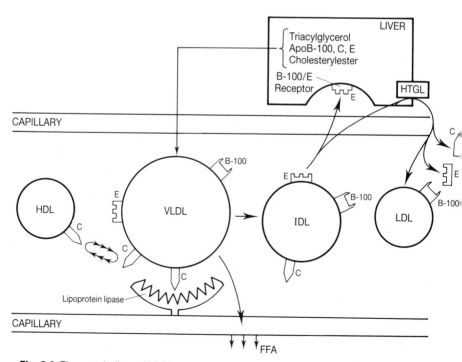

Fig. 8.6 The metabolism of VLDL

bind to LDL receptors in the hepatocyte surface and be cleared by endocytosis. This route accounts for up to 50 per cent of the IDL in humans. Alternatively the IDL may undergo further hydrolysis under the action of the HTGL bound to the hepatocyte membrane. This results in a loss of apoproteins C and E to HDL and the production of a cholesterylester-rich, low density lipoprotein (which contains a single molecule of apoB-100 as virtually its only apoprotein). *In vivo* it appears that larger VLDL particles enriched in apoE are quickly metabolised and endocytosed as IDL, while smaller VLDL particles are metabolized more slowly through to LDL.

Cholesterol-rich lipoproteins

Low density lipoproteins (LDL)

Low density lipoprotein is the primary cholesterol transport particle in the circulation, with cholesterylester 35–45 per cent and free cholesterol a further 6–15 per cent by weight. It serves as a cholesterol donor to both peripheral tissues and the liver, with the liver accounting for greater than 50 per cent of the total LDL uptake. The removal of LDL by both the liver and extrahepatic tissues is via receptor-mediated endocytosis involving the apoB/E or LDL receptor (Fig. 8.7). This protein of 839 amino acids is anchored to the cell surface by a membrane-spanning region near its C-terminal. Part of the protein shows

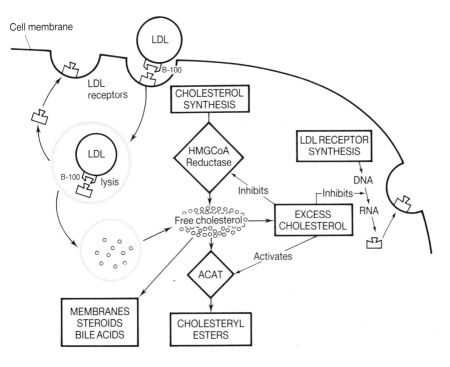

Fig. 8.7 Metabolism of LDL and cellular cholesterol homoeostasis

sequence homology with epidermal growth factor and the LDL-binding region, consisting of eight repeat sequences enriched in negatively-charged amino acids (especially cysteine) is located at the N-terminus. This negatively-charged region will bind the positively-charged region of the C-terminus of apoB-100. Since each LDL particle has only a single molecule of apoB-100, binding of LDL to the receptor is monovalent, i.e. one particle can bind to only one receptor.

Endocytosis of LDL results in the formation of an endosome with the LDL bound to its receptor inside the vesicle. Acidification of the endosome causes dissociation of the lipoprotein from the receptor and a separation such that many of the receptors are recycled to the cell surface, while the LDL is digested by lysosomal enzymes. Amino acids derived from hydrolysis of apoproteins enter the cellular amino acid pool.

Under normal conditions the free cholesterol concentration in the cell represents a balance between endogenous synthesis, exogenous LDL-derived cholesterol and esterification by ACAT. The increase of free cholesterol concentration as a result of hydrolysis of LDL-derived cholesterylester by the acid cholesterylester hydrolase has important consequences for cellular cholesterol metabolism, each of which attempts to restore the homoeostatic intracellular free cholesterol concentration (Table 8.3). Cholesterol or more likely an oxy-metabolite of cholesterol inhibits endogenous synthesis initially at the level of HMGCoA reductase and eventually by inhibition of transcription of the LDL receptor gene, leading to a reduction in the expression of the receptor at the cell surface. Hence uptake of exogenous cholesterol via LDL endocytosis is reduced. Finally, a rise in intracellular cholesterol activates the enzyme responsible for converting it to its storage ester form, ACAT. The converse of these actions occurs when the intracellular free cholesterol concentration falls.

High density lipoproteins (HDL)

The cholesterol content of cells is tightly regulated by the processes described above. Whereas VLDL and hence LDL transport cholesterol away from the liver to extrahepatic tissues, HDL is thought to play an important role in the removal of cholesterol from cells and mediating its transfer back to the liver, the process of reverse cholesterol transport (Fig. 8.8). This process is of utmost importance since the liver is the principal route of excretion of cholesterol from the body and

Table 8.3 The effect of the concentration of intracellular free cholesterol on cellular cholesterol metabolism and the expression of LDL receptors

Concentration of intracellular free cholesterol	LDL receptor synthesis	Receptor-mediated LDL uptake	HMGCoA reductase activity	ACAT activity
Low	↑	↑	↑	↓
High	↓	↓	↓	↑

the absence of HDL, seen in patients with Tangier disease leads to cholesterol accumulation in extrahepatic tissues.

Nascent HDL are secreted primarily by the liver and intestine as disc-shaped particles consisting of a phospholipid bilayer containing free cholesterol and apoproteins AI, AII and a little E. These discoidal particles interact with extrahepatic cells probably via a specific receptor (likely to be for apoAI) and accept free cholesterol from the plasma membrane down a concentration gradient. There is evidence that in some cells cholesterol is removed from an intracellular store and that in such cells the HDL enters the cell, accepts free cholesterol from this internal store and returns to the plasma membrane by retroendocytosis. Since cholesterol is stored as its ester the first step in reverse cholesterol transport must be hydrolysis of the ester to free cholesterol which is accepted by HDL. Both of the two mechanisms described leads to the formation of a cholesterol-enriched particle. The action of the extracellular LCAT, activated by apoAI, converts the free cholesterol of HDL to cholesterylester which moves to the hydrophobic interior of the particle, causing a change in shape from a discoidal to a spherical particle (HDL$_3$). This is a very rapid process so that very little discoidal HDL is present in plasma and the conversion of HDL-cholesterol to its ester maintains the concentration gradient between the extrahepatic tissue and HDL. That this concentration gradient is important is shown in patients with severe liver disease, where LCAT production is markedly decreased and erythrocytes become loaded with free cholesterol with a concomitant rise in plasma phospholipid and free cholesterol. *In vitro*, HDL$_3$ can also serve as an acceptor of free cholesterol from cholesterol-loaded cells and here too this free cholesterol is esterified by the apoAI-activated LCAT. The further incorporation of cholesterylester reduces the particle density to that of HDL$_2$. It is likely that this process also occurs *in vivo* since both HDL$_3$ and HDL$_2$ species

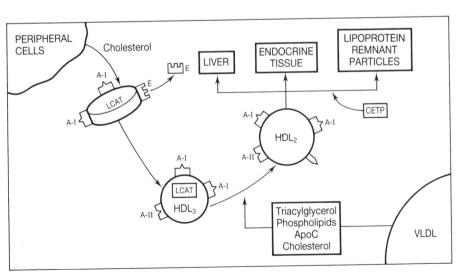

Fig. 8.8 The metabolism of HDL

can be isolated from human plasma. While some of the HDL may interact with hepatic receptors, it appears that much of the cholesterylester of HDL is not transported directly to the liver but is transferred to a liver-destined lipoprotein such as IDL, CMR and possibly LDL by the action of a cholesterylester transfer protein (CETP). As HDL_3 becomes loaded with cholesterylester the particles lose most of their apoE and gain more apoAII and the formation of HDL_2 is associated with the transfer of free cholesterol, triglyceride, phospholipids and apoC from the triglyceride-rich lipoproteins (VLDL and CM). LCAT action appears to facilitate apoprotein movement to and from chylomicrons. As mentioned earlier, movement of cholesterol from cell to HDL is down a concentration gradient and it is likely that this is the norm *in vivo*. However, it is possible that cholesterol might move from HDL to the cell if the cellular concentration is low and there is some evidence that HDL might donate free cholesterol to steroidogenic tissues.

Lipoprotein(a) (Lp(a))

In 1960 Berg described a broad class of lipoproteins with pre-β-electrophoretic mobility which consisted of LDL in which apoB-100 was linked to a glycoprotein (apoprotein(a)) via one or two disulphide bridges. The heterogeneity of this lipoprotein was due to differences in the protein: lipid ratio, apoB : apo(a) ratio, apo(a) polymorphism and its degree of glycosylation. There was also heterogeneity in its lipid composition and in particular the cholesterylester and triglyceride content of the particle core.

Apoprotein(a) is a glycoprotein containing up to 30 per cent by weight of carbohydrate and shows structural similarity to plasminogen with a variable number (15–40) of kringle 4 domain regions giving rise to size polymorphism (300–800 kDa). This size polymorphism is under the control of several alleles at the apo(a) gene locus on the long arm of chromosome 6.

Lp(a) is synthesized in the liver and although cholesterylester-rich and triglyceride-rich species are present in the plasma the normal physiological role of these particles, if any, is not known. It may be that Lp(a) can deliver cholesterol to sites not accessible to the LDL pathway. The plasma concentration of Lp(a) is strongly controlled by genetic factors and varies markedly from 0–100 mg/dl. From epidemiological studies it is claimed that a concentration of Lp(a) in excess of 30 mg/dl is an independent risk factor for coronary heart disease and Lp(a) has been demonstrated in atherosclerotic plaques. It is possible that its similarity to plasminogen might enable it to compete with plasminogen for binding to fibrin or the plasminogen receptor, causing an increase in plasminogen and promoting thrombogenesis by inhibiting thrombolytic mechanisms.

The interactions of lipoproteins with their receptors are essential for lipid homoeostasis. Genetically-determined abnormalities which give rise to overproduction and/or impaired removal of any particular lipoprotein present clinically as primary lipidaemias (Table 8.4).

Table 8.4 Genetic/metabolic causes of primary hyperlipidaemias

Disease	Primary disorder	Metabolic disorder	CHD risk	Pancreatitis
Common hypercholesterolaemia	Multiple genetic/environmental factor	LDL over-production and decreased LDL catabolism	+	
Familial combined hyperlipidaemia	Unknown	Over-production of VLDL apoB-100 and/or LDL apo B-100	+ +	
Familial hypercholesterolaemia	At least 190 mutations causing impaired LDLR function	LDL over-production and impaired LDL catabolism	+ + + +	
Remnant (Type III) hyperlipidaemia	Coexistence of non-functional apoE isoforms with genetic or acquired disorder of VLDL/LDL metabolism	Impaired conversion of remnant particle to LDL	+ + +	?
Familial hypertriglyceridaemia	Unknown	Increased VLDL production and/or decreased VLDL catabolism	?	+ +
Chylomicronaemia syndrome	Deficiency of lipoprotein lipase or its essential cofactor apoCII	Impaired clearance of CM. Sometimes secondary impairment of VLDL removal		+ +

Atherosclerosis

Atherosclerosis is the most common lethal disease in western populations. It has no single obvious cause and the major risk factors, hyperlipidaemia, hypertension and cigarette smoking, are not related in any simple way.

Atherosclerosis is a disease of the large and medium-sized arteries in which the intima of the arterial wall is thickened by development of fibrous tissue and the accumulation of lipid. Clinical manifestation of the disease mostly results from lesions in the aorta and arteries supplying the heart, brain and lower limbs. The lesions can result in a range of severe diseases caused by gradual occlusion of the artery, sudden occlusion or haemorrhage (Fig. 8.9). The most characteristic feature of developing atherosclerosis is the fibrous plaque, an area of intimal thickening which protrudes into the lumen of the artery. The thickening consists of an accumulation of fibrous connective tissue containing smooth muscle cells loaded with cholesterylester and forming an overlay deposit of extracellular cholesterylester and cell debris. Complicated lesions, which are the main cause of occlusion of the artery, develop from the fibrous plaques.

Pathogenesis

This is summarized in Fig. 8.10. Initiation (associated with the risk factors mentioned above) is currently thought to result from injury to the endothelial layer which normally forms the luminal face of the vessel wall. A damaged endothelium leads to deposition and aggregation of platelets at the site of injury with subsequent release of mitogenic agents such as platelet-derived growth factor from platelets, macrophages and the endothelium itself, which stimulate smooth muscle cell proliferation. The initial aggregation of platelets at the injured site may be promoted by an imbalance in the local PGI_2/TXA_2 ratio (Chapter 1). The stimulated smooth muscle cells are able to synthesize collagen, microfibrillar components of elastic tissue and the large amounts of glycosaminoglycans characteristic of the atherosclerotic plaque. The damaged endothelium also shows increased permeability to plasma components which raise the intimal LDL concentration and releases factors which are chemoattractant to circulating monocytes. Thus cholesterol loading of smooth muscle cells and monocyte-derived macrophages will occur. As the proportion of the lipid-rich debris in the plaque increases, ruptures or tears in the fibromuscular cap ensue with further platelet adhesion and aggregation and

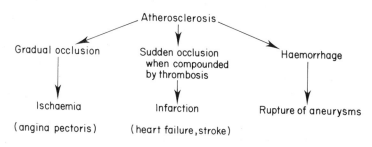

Fig. 8.9 Clinical consequences of atherosclerosis

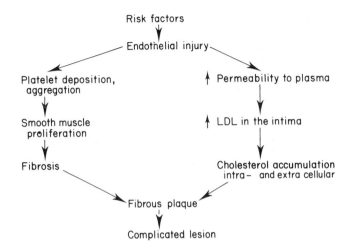

Fig. 8.10 Pathogenesis of atherosclerosis

narrowing of the arterial lumen. Once the plaque has formed it disturbs normal blood flow, increasing the likelihood of further damage and thrombus formation. Examination of complicated lesions of occluded arteries reveal masses of aggregated platelets associated with fibrin, cell debris and large amounts of crystalline cholesterol.

Role of LDL cholesterol in atherogenesis

Whilst a large body of evidence correlates elevated LDL-cholesterol levels with the occurrence of atherosclerosis it was not until the elegant studies of Goldstein and Brown with fibroblasts *in vitro* that a mechanism for the link could be advanced.

The receptor-mediated (high affinity) route for binding and uptake of the LDL particle has already been described (p. 123). The particular importance of this route is that it allows the cell to regulate the uptake of LDL-cholesterol, the endogenous synthesis of cholesterol and the storage as cholesterylester according to its needs. A feature of critical importance is that over-accumulation of cholesterol in the cell results in decreased receptor number and thus a decreased LDL-cholesterol entry rate. At very low concentrations of LDL this pathway accounts for virtually all of the cholesterol input to cells and achieves a precise control of cellular cholesterol metabolism. However, all cells also have the capacity to take in LDL by a receptor-independent, low affinity process resembling non-specific endocytosis. Here the rate of LDL entry is proportional to its concentration up to high values. Both processes result in degradation of the internalized LDL and accumulation of intracellular cholesterol, but only the receptor-mediated entry is self-regulatory. Accumulation of intracellular cholesterol shuts off entry by the receptor-mediated process but does not affect entry by the receptor-independent route. Thus at high concentrations of LDL a large part of cholesterol entry to cells is via the uncontrolled low affinity process. Both of these routes have now been shown to operate *in vivo* in animals and man. In normal individuals the receptor-mediated route accounts for 33 to 60 per cent of whole body LDL catabolism. Studies in pigs, rabbits and rats show that the organ making the greatest contribution to whole body LDL catabolism is the liver, with more than 50 per cent of the total rate. In terms of degradation rate per g of tissue liver is also the most active tissue. The contribution of the receptor-mediated pathway to LDL breakdown in liver was almost 70 per cent in normal lipaemic rats, but in animals made hypercholesterolaemic the contribution of the receptor-mediated process was reduced to 39 per cent of the total. Thus *in vivo*, as well as *in vitro*, the receptor-mediated route is most prominent in LDL catabolism only at lower LDL concentrations. At elevated LDL concentrations *in vivo* the resulting down-regulation of the high affinity receptor pathway ensures that the receptor-independent process contributes an increasingly greater proportion to total LDL catabolism.

The importance of the high affinity receptor-mediated pathway of LDL uptake and metabolism is amply demonstrated in the case of homozygotes for the genetic disorder familial hypercholesterolaemia. These individuals have no functional high affinity receptors and as a result catabolism of LDL can proceed only by the receptor-independent mechanism. This results in a decreased fractional clearance rate of LDL and consequently an extremely high plasma concentration of LDL cholesterol. The occurrence of atherosclerosis in these individuals is high, with the average age for development of myocardial infarction being 20 years.

Goldstein and Brown have proposed that the receptor-mediated and receptor-independent pathways are antagonistic in their influence on atherogenesis. Thus the former functions to protect against the disease whilst the latter predisposes to it. In normal animals and man high plasma concentrations of LDL channel LDL catabolism through the receptor-independent pathway and would therefore be associated with atherogenesis.

Most body cells do not obtain LDL directly from plasma but from the interstitial fluid, that is, the ultrafiltrate of plasma through the endothelium. The concentration of LDL in this fluid is around one-tenth that of the plasma. Studies of human cells *in vitro* have shown that the maximal percentage contribution of the high affinity receptor-mediated pathway to the catabolism of LDL occurs at an LDL-cholesterol concentration of around 0.07 mmol. At higher concentrations the cells' need for cholesterol is exceeded, resulting in down-regulation of receptors whilst the receptor-independent process is allowing a greater input to occur. Therefore for maximal efficiency of LDL receptor function the plasma LDL cholesterol concentration should be around 0.7 mmol. This happens to be the level of LDL-cholesterol observed in plasma of normal human neonates and animals not subject to atherosclerosis. At this concentration any plasma LDL-cholesterol leaking in to the artery wall through areas of damage would be removed efficiently by smooth muscle cells via the high affinity pathway and used for the normal growth requirements of the cell. But even at the mean concentration of LDL cholesterol prevailing in 'normal' western populations (around 3 mM) the load of LDL-cholesterol presented to smooth muscle cells and tissue macrophages when plasma leaks into the artery wall is sufficient to exceed the clearance capacity of the receptor-mediated process. LDL is therefore taken up by the receptor-independent route leading to an uncontrolled accumulation of cholesterylester in excess of the cells' needs. The smooth muscle cells take on the appearance of the foam cells characteristic of atheroma. Further accumulation of cholesterylester causes toxicity and cell death, resulting in the lipid deposits and cell debris that comprise a large part of the fibrous plaque of atherosclerosis. Thus, as a result of dietary and other stresses the increased dietary input of cholesterol in western man exceeds the normal catabolic capacity of the body (mainly the liver) resulting in raised plasma LDL and increased atherogenesis.

Oxidized LDL

While there seems little doubt that the monocyte-derived macrophage is the major precursor of foam cells in the fatty streak and atherosclerotic lesion, the accumulation of LDL-derived cholesterol by these cells presents a paradox. Macrophages express the LDL-receptor but, as was described above, this expression is under the control of the intracellular free cholesterol concentration and the receptor number is down regulated as the cells accumulate cholesterol. It also has not been possible to generate foam cells *in vitro* using high concentrations of LDL as the cholesterol donor. However, modification of LDL, particularly neutralization of the ε-amino groups of lysine residues of apoB, leads to a species of lipoprotein which is taken up by macrophages at a much greater rate than native LDL via a specific, saturable receptor. Original *in vitro* experiments used chemically-modified LDL (e.g. acetyl LDL) but many cells, including endothelial cells and even macrophages themselves are capable of oxidizing LDL to a modified form recognized by this scavenger receptor. Unlike the LDL receptor these scavenger receptors, which are expressed as the monocyte differentiates into a tissue macrophage, appear not to be down-regulated by accumulation of cholesterol in the cell. Furthermore, the properties of oxidized LDL (Table 8.5) indicate that it is potentially more atherogenic than native LDL in a number of ways, as outlined in Fig. 8.11.

The properties described in Table 8.5 are those of LDL which has undergone major oxidation so that it is no longer recognized by the LDL receptor. Such a species of LDL may be produced in the subendothelium but it is unlikely to occur in the circulation because of the antioxidants present (e.g. vitamin E, HDL, erythrocytes etc.). However, LDL may undergo a mild oxidation in the circulation giving rise to a minimally modified LDL (MM-LDL) where some of the fatty acids of the surface phospholipids are oxidized to reactive aldehydes but where the ε-amino group of lysine residues on apoprotein B are intact and the particle is still recognized by the apoB receptor on monocytes and endothelial cells. MM-LDL promotes the adhesion of circulating monocytes to the endothelium and their migration into the subendothelial space. MM-LDL also stimulates the release of cytokines from the endothelial cells including a monocyte chemotactic factor (MCP-1) which ensures the prolonged residence of the trapped monocytes and macrophage-colony stimulating factor (M-CSF) which promotes the differentiation of monocytes to macrophages and the expression of scavenger receptors on the macrophage surface. These monocyte-derived macrophages can now accumulate lipid from fully oxidized LDL (OX-LDL), in which the apoprotein B has been modified, via the non regulated scavenger receptors. Excessive accumulation of lipid leads to the formation of foam cells. These events are exacerbated by the cytotoxic properties of OX-LDL which cause damage to the endothelium, allowing further monocyte infiltration and platelet aggregation at the site of the damage.

There is increasing circumstantial evidence that processes akin to those described might occur *in vivo*. For instance, (i) immunocytochemical detection of OX-LDL in atherosclerotic lesions in rabbits; (ii) isolation of a species of LDL from human and rabbit lesions which is immunologically similar to OX-LDL; (iii) detection of autoantibodies to charge modified LDL in human and rabbit serum. Also, probucol, a drug known to have antioxidant properties inhibited

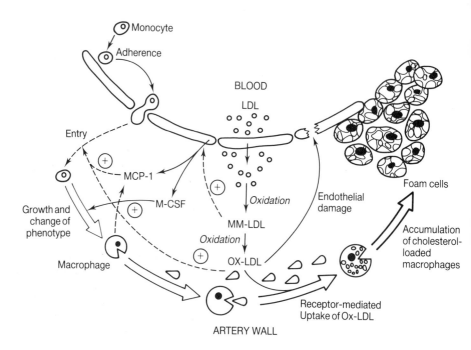

Fig. 8.11 A schematic outline of the oxidative modification hypothesis, showing the several ways in which oxidized low density lipoprotein (LDL) is potentially more atherogenic than native LDL. Monocytes, the major precursor for foam cells in the fatty streak, are shown adhering to the endothelium and then penetrating to the subendothelial space. Oxidized LDL can directly stimulate this by virtue of its lysolecithin content and lightly oxidized LDL (MM-LDL) can stimulate indirectly by increasing the release of MCP-1 from endothelial cells. Oxidized LDL is a ligand for the scavenger receptor that is expressed as the monocyte differentiates to a tissue macrophage and this leads to the accumulation of lipids in the developing foam cells. This monocyte/macrophage differentiation can be facilitated by the release of macrophage-colony stimulating factor (M-CSF) from endothelial cells under the influence of MM-LDL. Finally, oxidized LDL can induce endothelial damage and thus facilitate the atherogenic process by allowing entry of elements from the blood and by allowing adherence of platelets. Additional properties of oxidized LDL not shown here that may make it more atherogenic are the facts that it is immunogenic and that it interferes with the response of arteries to endothelial-derived relaxation factor (EDRF). Reproduced with permission Steinberg, D. Antioxidants and Atherosclerosis *Circulation Research* **84** (1991) 1420–25 copyright 1991 American Heart Association

Table 8.5   Properties of oxidized LDL

1. Chemotactic for circulating monocytes.
2. Inhibits the motility of resident macrophages.
3. Cytotoxic to cells in culture.
4. Stimulates the release of a chemotactic factor from endothelial cells in culture.
5. Stimulates release of colony stimulating factor and monocyte chemotactic factor from endothelial cells in culture.

atheroma formation in an animal model. Two cDNAs for human macrophage scavenger receptors have been cloned and show high amino acid sequence homology with two previously described bovine scavenger receptors. The receptor gene which is located on chromosome 8 in humans gave rise to receptors which endocytosed modified LDL when expressed in a continuous cell line. With antiserum to peptides derived from the deduced amino acid sequence, the scavenger receptor proteins were demonstrated histochemically in macrophages of atherosclerotic lesions.

Thus it seems likely that oxidation of LDL may well play a major role in atherogenesis but much more needs to be learned about the mechanism before making recommendations on how to combat it *in vivo*. Although cellular lipoxygenases and the superoxide anion have been implicated the precise oxidizing species is unknown. It may be that dietary changes will afford some protection. For instance, increased consumption of exogenous antioxidants such as β-carotene, vitamins C and E might raise an individual's oxygen scavenging potential. Also the nature of dietary fatty acids might have a protective role. The susceptibility of LDL to oxidation is related to the fatty acid composition of its phospholipid component, polyunsaturated fatty acids (PUFA) being more readily oxidized than monounsaturated fatty acids (MUFA). It is possible to increase the MUFA content of LDL by feeding diets low in PUFA and high in MUFA and thereby generate an oxidation-resistant LDL. However, such fanciful ideas await results from more basic research.

Treatment of hypercholesterolaemia

As described earlier, the homoeostatic concentration of cholesterol in the blood is a balance between input from the diet and endogenous synthesis, particularly in the liver, and excretion via the bile as neutral sterols and bile acids. Obviously a first approach to the treatment of hypercholesterolaemia would involve a reduction in the cholesterol content of the diet by switching to low fat foods accompanied by attempts to reduce body weight. This may prove quite successful for the mildly hypercholesterolaemic patient. However, in cases of marked hypercholesterolaemia, drug therapy may be required to reduce serum cholesterol towards the normal range. Two major classes of drug have been used with some success in humans: the bile acid binding resins and the statins.

Bile acid binding resins

The rationale for the use of bile acid binding resins (sequestrants) such as cholestyramine is 2-fold. Firstly, bile acids are required for the formation of micelles from which dietary fat is absorbed in the intestine. Thus, after administration the resin complexes with the bile acids and reduces absorption of dietary fat including cholesterol. Secondly, the resins interrupt the enterohepatic cycling of bile acids and increase their excretion in the faeces. Under normal circumstances approximately 95 per cent of the bile acids secreted into the intestine are reabsorbed in the terminal ileum and only a small fraction of the total bile acid pool is lost each day. Interruption of the cycle results in increased hepatic synthesis of bile acids from endogenous cholesterol. Initially the free cholesterol concentration of the liver falls as it is used for bile acid synthesis and this reduction causes an increase in hepatic LDL receptor synthesis and consequent increased clearance of LDL. Another consequence of a fall in hepatic free cholesterol is that endogenous cholesterol synthesis increases as the amount and activity of HMGCoAR rises and this may counteract the cholesterol-lowering action of the bile acid binding resin. The postulated mechanism of bile acid sequestration is outlined in Fig. 8.12.

Statins (HMGCoAR inhibitors)

Since the liver synthesizes almost one gram of cholesterol daily, inhibition of *de novo* synthesis represents an attractive way of lowering plasma cholesterol. Two compounds, compactin and mevinolin, isolated from culture broths of *Penicillium*

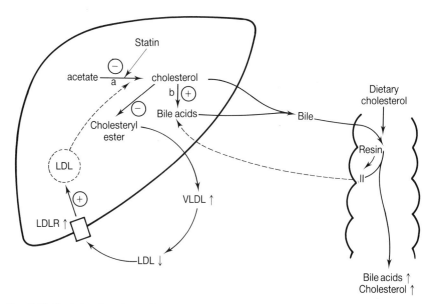

Fig. 8.12 Postulated actions of bile acid sequestrants and HMGCoA reductase inhibitors of LDL metabolism. a: HMGCoA reductase; b: cholesterol 7α-hydroxylase; LDLR: LDL receptor

citrinum and *Aspergillus terreus* respectively, are both competitive inhibitors of HMGCoAR and have given rise to a family of inhibitors known as the statins. The structure of these compounds resembles that of the half-reduced intermediate of the HMGCoAR reaction and may be the basis of their inhibitory action. Administration of the drugs as their inactive, precursor lactone ensured efficient first-pass removal by the liver such that little is found in extra hepatic tissues. Hydrolysis of the lactone produces the active hydroxy-acid which binds competitively to the active site of the enzyme. Many of the current synthetic statins are free hydroxy-acids but are also cleared by a rapid first-pass effect governed primarily by their water solubility. This tissue selectivity is particularly important, since inhibition of cholesterol synthesis in tissues other than liver, especially nervous tissue and those such as adrenal cortex which are responsible for steroid hormone synthesis, may be undesirable.

The inhibition of hepatic cholesterol synthesis reduces VLDL synthesis by limiting cholesterol for export and increases the number of high affinity LDL receptors on the hepatic cell surface. LDL catabolism is thus also increased (Fig. 8.12). The statins are currently the most effective drugs for reducing LDL cholesterol levels. In cases of particularly high hypercholesterolaemia, where the statin alone does not achieve a sufficient reduction, a combination of a statin and a bile acid binding resin is likely to be effective. Statin therapy would of course produce no effect in homozygous familial hypercholesterolaemia patients with an absence of or defective LDL receptor. It is also important to mention that, whereas statins are extremely effective at reducing LDL cholesterol, there is as yet no clinical evidence that such an effect reduces the morbidity and mortality associated with coronary heart disease, in contrast to bile acid binding resins.

9

Calcium metabolism

The body contains about 1 kg of calcium (Fig. 9.1), the majority of which is present in bone as hydroxyapatite. Although quantitatively much smaller, the calcium pools within the soft tissues and the extracellular fluid (ECF) are critical to a wide range of metabolic processes. The importance of these functions is reflected in the tight control of ECF calcium. This is achieved through the regulation of calcium transport between intestine, bone and kidney by a number of hormones and physicochemical processes.

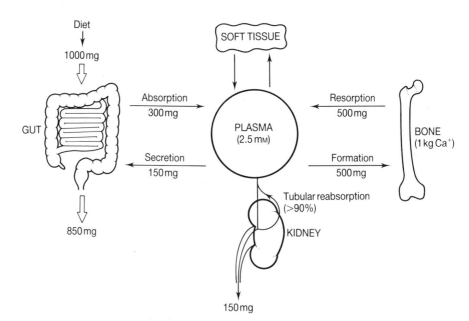

Fig. 9.1 Daily calcium flux in calcium compartments during normal calcium homoeostasis in the adult human (40 mg = 1 mmol calcium)

The control of extracellular fluid calcium

ECF calcium homoeostasis is maintained by the integrated effects of parathyroid hormone (PTH) and 1,25 dihydroxy vitamin D (1,25(OH)$_2$D) on the gut, kidney and bone (Fig. 9.2). Both hormones act to regulate the fluxes of calcium between these three target organs and the ECF so that under normal circumstances the calcium concentration varies by less than 5 per cent. This also ensures that calcium balance is zero: the amount of calcium lost from the body in urine and sweat is exactly balanced by the net amount absorbed by the gut.

Calcium is present in the ECF as free ionized calcium (50 per cent), a component bound to protein (40 per cent), mainly albumin and a diffusible fraction (10 per cent) made up of calcium salts such as citrate and lactate. It is the ionized component which is of physiological importance and the focus of homoeostatic control. The protein-bound calcium is of practical significance since increases or decreases in serum albumin will respectively increase or decrease total serum calcium (normal range 2.2–2.6 mmol/l). Since measurement of ionized calcium is not available routinely in hospital laboratories the total serum calcium must be 'corrected' for changes in albumin:

Corrected calcium = measured calcium + 0.02 (40 − albumin) mmol/l

where serum albumin is expressed in g/l.

Short-term changes in serum calcium from minute-to-minute over the range 1.9–2.9 mmol/l are regulated by PTH action on the labile calcium pool in bone

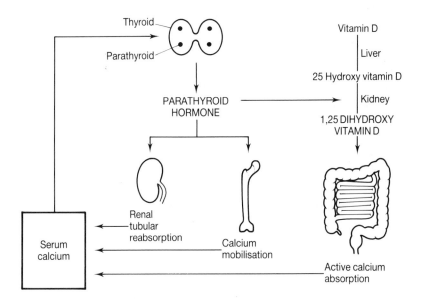

Fig. 9.2 PTH – Vitamin D cycle

and calcium excretion/reabsorption by the kidney. Longer term adaptation over hours to days depends on the effect of PTH on $1,25(OH)_2D$ synthesis and secondarily on intestinal calcium absorption.

The PTH – vitamin D endocrine system

The way in which the actions of PTH and vitamin D are integrated is fundamental to an understanding of calcium homoeostasis (Fig. 9.2).

Parathyroid hormone

PTH is synthesized in the endoplasmic reticulum of the parathyroid glands as an initial translation product of 115 amino acids (pre-pro-PTH). The leader sequence of 25 amino acids is essential for translocating the peptide to the endoplasmic reticulum and through the cisternal space. It is cleaved to a 90 amino acid peptide (pro-PTH) prior to entry into the Golgi apparatus and then again to the mature 1–84 peptide in the secretory granules. Only amino acids 1–34 are required for biological activity. Intact PTH is further cleaved after secretion with the result that immunogenic, but biologically inert, fragments are present in the circulation. This has presented problems with immunoassays for PTH but these have now been resolved by the introduction of two site assays which measure the intact 1–84 peptide.

PTH secretion is exquisitely sensitive to deviations from an individual's 'set point' calcium: a fall is counteracted by an increase, and a rise by a decrease, in secretion. PTH acts alone on the renal tubule to regulate calcium and phosphate excretion and to modulate the production of $1,25(OH)_2D$. Together with $1,25(OH)_2D$ it regulates calcium and phosphate exchange between bone and ECF.

PTH action at a cellular level

Parathyroid hormone activates target cells such as those in the proximal renal tubule via stimulation of adenylate cyclase and the synthesis of cAMP (see Chapter 1; Fig. 1.8). Binding of PTH to its receptor on the cell surface activates guanyl nucleotide binding proteins (G-proteins) in the cell membrane. The G-proteins are made up of α, β and γ polypeptide chains and cycle between an active GTP-binding form and an inactive GDP-binding form. When PTH activates the receptor, GTP exchanges for GDP on the α chain and causes its dissociation from the β and γ chains. This in turn stimulates the activity of adenylate cyclase, situated on the cytosolic surface of the cell membrane, which catalyses the production of cAMP. This is the major second messenger within the cell which acts through a series of protein kinases to regulate intracellular phosphorylation that in turn results in expression of the effect of PTH on the cell. In the proximal renal tubule this includes the excretion of phosphate and stimulation of the 25(OH)D, 1α-hydroxylase system resulting in the production of $1,25(OH)_2D$.

PTH may also activate target cells through a cAMP-independent mechanism by coupling to a receptor whose activation leads to the hydrolysis of phosphatidyl inositol 4, 5 bisphosphate (PIP_2) by a specific phosphodiesterase (Chapter 1; Figs. 1.9 and 1.10). This leads to the formation of diacylglycerol (DAG) and inositol trisphosphate (IP_3) which act as intracellular messengers. IP_3 diffuses into the cell cytosol to release calcium from the endoplasmic reticulum, thus activating calmodulin dependent protein kinases (Chapter 1; Fig. 1.11). This in turn catalyses the phosphorylation of proteins which are responsible for the initial phase of the cellular response. DAG, acting within the plane of the plasma membrane, activates protein kinase C, which seems important in sustaining the cellular response to activation.

Vitamin D

Vitamin D is a secosteroid of which cholecalciferol (D_3) and ergocalciferol (D_2) are the most important compounds. For practical purposes they can be regarded as being interchangeable in man.

Dietary sources and cutaneous synthesis

Vitamin D is obtained either from the diet (D_2 or D_3) or from endogenous synthesis in skin (D_3). Dairy produce, eggs and oily fish are the main sources of D_3 whilst the fortification of margarine with D_2 from plant sources is probably quantitatively the most valuable. Ultraviolet light causes the non-enzymic photolysis of epidermal 7-dehydrocholesterol to pre-vitamin D_3 which then slowly isomerases to vitamin D_3. In the absence of cutaneous synthesis the dietary requirement to avoid clinical deficiency is of the order of 2.5 μg/day for an adult and 10 μg/day for a child.

Hepatic hydroxylation

Vitamin D from cutaneous synthesis or from upper small intestinal absorption is transported to the liver bound to a specific α-globulin (D-binding protein), albumin and lipoproteins. Here it is 25-hydroxylated by a microsomal mixed function oxidase which requires NADPH, molecular oxygen and magnesium for its regulation. 25(OH)D is two to five times more potent than parent D in terms of calcium absorption and bone resorption but several orders of magnitude less potent than 1,25(OH)$_2$D. Hydroxylation of 25(OH)D is not tightly product-inhibited and high circulating concentrations may be found where there is substrate excess, for example vitamin D overdosage. 25(OH)D is the major circulating form of vitamin D and may also be stored in fat and liver.

Renal hydroxylation

The most important step in the activation of vitamin D occurs in the proximal convoluted and proximal straight tubules of the kidney where 25(OH)D is converted to 1,25(OH)$_2$D by a mitochondrial mixed function monooxygenase. This 1α-hydroxylase is predominantly regulated by PTH and intracellular phosphate concentrations and by a lesser extent by calcium, calcitonin, growth hormone, oestrogens and prolactin. It is strongly product-inhibited and as 1α-hydroxylase activity decreases there is a reciprocal increase in the activity of the renal 24-hydroxylase with synthesis of $24,25(OH)_2D$. Whether this latter metabolite has a significant physiological role is at present uncertain.

$1,25(OH)_2D$ is the major biologically active metabolite of vitamin D, with important effects on gut and bone. Although $1,25(OH)_2D$ may suppress PTH secretion it is uncertain whether this is a physiological or a pharmacological effect.

Effects of PTH and 1,25(OH)₂D on intestine, kidney and bone

Intestinal calcium and phosphate absorption

Calcium and phosphate are absorbed by an active transport process in the duodenum and jejunum and by facilitated diffusion in the distal intestine. Although the rate of absorption is most active in the proximal intestine, the major portion of the dietary calcium intake is absorbed in distal segments because of their greater length and surface area. The mechanism by which absorption occurs is uncertain but both processes are stimulated by $1,25(OH)_2D$. Although $1,25(OH)_2D$ stimulates the synthesis of calcium-binding proteins by intestinal cells they appear after calcium absorption has increased and persist after the effect has waned. PTH has no direct effect on intestinal absorption but regulates this process according to the needs of calcium homoeostasis through its effect on the renal synthesis of $1,25(OH)_2D$. This process of adaptation, which takes from hours to days to reach a new steady state, links changes in ECF calcium to compensatory changes in calcium absorption which act to restore homoeostasis. The mechanisms by which $1,25(OH)_2D$ regulate absorption are uncertain. The pathological causes of altered calcium absorption are shown in Table 9.1.

Renal tubular calcium and phosphate reabsorption

Under the influence of PTH, and without apparent involvement of $1,25(OH)_2D$, the kidney regulates the reabsorption of calcium and phosphate independently one from the other. This contrasts with their co-transport in intestine and bone and places the kidney at the centre of calcium and phosphate regulation.

Calcium and magnesium

More than 95 per cent of the non-protein bound calcium filtered at the glomerulus will subsequently be reabsorbed by the renal tubules. The bulk of this reabsorption, in the proximal nephron, is by hormone-independent transport although PTH regulates the critical last stage of distal reabsorption. In general terms the filtered load of calcium just exceeds the maximum capacity of tubular reabsorption (which is set by PTH) so that as the filtered load increases then so does its excretion, while the converse occurs as calcium load falls.

Table 9.1 Pathological causes of altered calcium absorption

Increased absorption
(a) Increased 1,25(OH)$_2$D
Increased amounts of substrate: vitamin D overdosage
Enhanced 1α-hydroxylase activity: hyperparathyroidism
Extrarenal production: sarcoidosis and other granulomata
T- and B-cell lymphomas

(b) Increased calcium availability
Increased calcium intake, low phosphate or phytate diets

Decreased absorption
(a) Decreased 1,25(OH)$_2$D
Decreased amounts of substrate: vitamin D deficiency
Decreased 1α-hydroxylase activity: chronic renal failure
Reduced PTH secretion: hypoparathyroidism suppression due to hypercalcaemia
PTH resistance

(b) Decreased calcium transport
Intestinal disease: coeliac disease (duodenum, jejunum)
Crohn's disease (ileum)
Low calcium, high phosphate/phytate diets
Drugs: corticosteroids, sodium fluoride

In the proximal renal tubule, calcium and magnesium appear to be reabsorbed passively down a concentration gradient through the tight junctions. The driving force is the reabsorption of sodium, which occurs by a number of mechanisms. These include specific co-transporters in the luminal membrane, a neutral transport which includes a sodium–hydrogen exchanger, isolated entry of sodium into cells and the passive movement through tight junctions and lateral spaces. Solute transport, particularly that of sodium, creates an osmotic gradient down which water moves passively, thereby creating the gradient for calcium and magnesium reabsorption. This means that the delivery of calcium and magnesium to the distal nephron will change whenever proximal reabsorption of sodium and water is altered. These mechanisms underline the observation that calcium excretion is increased during natriuresis and decreased during sodium conservation.

The tight junctions of the proximal tubule are relatively impermeable to magnesium and proportionately less is reabsorbed by comparison with calcium; hence its concentration rises in more distal portions of the proximal tubule. Such absorption that occurs does so across the tight junctions, similar to that of calcium.

In the early diluting segment, calcium and magnesium are both strongly reabsorbed. The positive luminal potential provides the driving force for transport through the tight junctions, presumably coupled to active transport across the basolateral membrane.

In the late diluting segment and more distal portions of the nephron calcium enters cells passively and is actively transported across the basolateral membrane into the peritubular space. PTH enhances this process by a cAMP-mediated increase in the calcium permeability of the luminal membrane. As ECF calcium increases, two independent mechanisms act to restore homoeostasis. First, PTH secretion will be suppressed and this will reduce the stimulus to distal tubular calcium reabsorption. Second, a rise in the serum calcium will increase the filtered load which will deliver more calcium to a relatively impermeable distal tubule. This results in more calcium being excreted and homoeostasis being restored. Converse changes occur when ECF calcium falls.

The other stimulus to altered calcium reabsorption which is important in clinical medicine is the effect of changes in ECF volume. As ECF volume expands there will be an increase in GFR and reduced sodium reabsorption in the proximal tubule. This will increase calcium delivery to the distal nephron and therefore tend to augment calcium excretion. However, providing that parathyroid function is normal, any tendency to hypocalcaemia will be offset by an increase in PTH secretion which will stimulate distal tubular calcium transport and offset the effects of decreased proximal reabsorption. Unfortunately there are a number of clinical situations where changes in ECF volume occur at times when parathyroid function is compromised. Under these circumstances calcium homoeostasis may be jeopardized by changes in ECF volume.

Phosphate

The filtered load of phosphate slightly exceeds the overall maximal tubular reabsorption so that phosphate spills into the urine. Phosphate is actively reabsorbed in the proximal tubule through a sodium–phosphate co-transporter across the brush border and facilitated passive transport at the basolateral membrane. PTH, acting through the intracellular generation of cAMP in the early portions of the proximal tubule, lowers the transport capacity of phosphate and also water and other solutes. In the later portions of the proximal tubule there is an inhibitory effect of PTH which seems to be specific to phosphate. More distal portions of the nephron appear relatively impermiant to phosphate since increased delivery out of the proximal tubule results in increased phosphaturia.

Renal mechanisms in the independent control of calcium and phosphate homoeostasis

Hypocalcaemia stimulates the secretion of PTH which in turn increases the entry of calcium and phosphate into the ECF from bone and intestine. However, the renal effect of PTH ensures that whilst calcium is reabsorbed, phosphate will be excreted. The result is a net increase in ECF calcium but phosphate will remain unchanged.

Hypophosphataemia stimulates the renal 1α-hydroxylase with a consequent increase in $1,25(OH)_2D$ and enhanced calcium and phosphate absorption from the intestine and probably increases calcium and phosphate transport from bone. The enhanced delivery of calcium to the ECF will suppress PTH secretion (assuming the presence of pure hypophosphataemia) with the consequence that the renal tubular reabsorption of phosphate will be enhanced but the increased filtered load of calcium will be eliminated.

In combined hypocalcaemia and hypophosphataemia calcium will be retained as described above, but as the ECF concentration rises the drive to PTH will diminish progressively. As the secondary hyperparathyroidism subsides there will be a progressive rise in the threshold for phosphate reabsorption so that phosphate will then be retained and the hypophosphataemia corrected.

The opposite changes operate in hypercalcaemia. Hyperphosphataemia in contrast, will tend to elevate the ECF Ca × P product which is normally near its solubility limit. This will lead to deposition of calcium phosphate in bone and soft tissues with a fall in the serum calcium which will stimulate PTH. This will inhibit distal tubular phosphate reabsorption so that the excess phosphate will be lost in the urine and homoeostasis restored. The major causes of altered calcium excretion are shown in Table 9.2.

Table 9.2   Altered excretion of calcium

Decreased calcium excretion
  Reduced filtered load due to hypocalcaemia
  Malabsorption of calcium from intestinal disease
  Increased tubular reabsorption (PTH, PTHrP)
  Increased proximal tubular sodium reabsorption (ECF depletion)

  Thiazide diuretics

Increased calcium excretion
  Increased filtered load due to hypercalcaemia
  Increased intestinal calcium absorption
  Renal leak of calcium (renal stone disease)
  Reduced levels of PTH

  ECF volume expansion, loop diuretics

Contribution of bone to calcium and phosphate homoeostasis

Two distinct processes must be considered in any description of the role of the skeleton in calcium homoeostasis. The first, regulated by PTH and $1,25(OH)_2D$ is the exchange of soluble calcium salts between a labile pool in bone and the ECF. This process involves the cells lining the bone surface and the osteocytes lying in the cannalicular space. The second process, where the mechanical integrity of bone is maintained over time through a regular cycle of bone remodelling, involves osteoclastic resorption and osteoblastic formation. Under normal circumstances the two components of remodelling are tightly coupled so that the amount of bone resorbed is exactly balanced by the bone formed. Calcium is therefore 'recycled' within the bone microenvironment without distortion of calcium homoeostasis. However, at times of stress when normal exchange mechanisms are exhausted there may be net bone resorption with destruction of mineralized bone in an attempt to maintain ECF calcium homoeostasis. A number of common diseases often lead to this pathological state of affairs. It is therefore important that the inter-relationship between calcium exchange, bone remodelling and calcium homoeostasis is clearly understood.

Calcium exchange between bone and ECF

Within the apparently solid structure of both cortical and trabecular bone there are bone cells (osteocytes) lying within fluid (bone ECF) filled cannalicular spaces (Fig. 9.3). Bone ECF is separated from bulk ECF by an intact layer of cells (lining cells) which are probably of the osteoblast lineage and are in physical continuity with the osteocyte network. Bulk ECF is supersaturated with calcium by comparison with bone ECF so that there is a tendency for calcium to diffuse down a concentration gradient into bone. Although this system is difficult to study, it is known that the bone lining cells have receptors for PTH and there are a number of mechanisms by which calcium might move out of bone into the bulk ECF in response to the need to maintain homoeostasis. Cells of the osteoblast lineage are effective producers of acid and this would be a way of increasing the solubility of bone mineral and therefore the calcium content of bone ECF. Transfer of calcium out of bone through the lining cells might occur either by diffusion or by calcium pumps, both of which might be modulated by PTH or other hormonal influences. It is clear that large quantities of calcium exchange between bulk and bone ECF and far exceed those moved by bone remodelling.

Bone remodelling

By its very nature, the skeleton is subjected to repeated physical stress. It is perhaps to be expected that mechanisms exist whereby bone can be

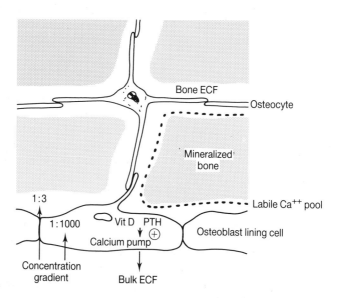

Fig. 9.3 Role of bone in calcium homoeostatis

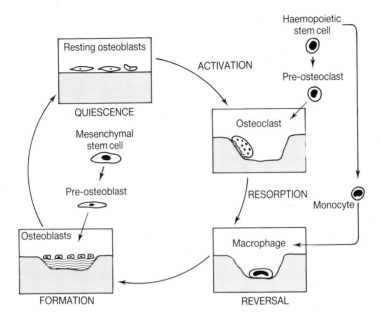

Fig. 9.4 Bone remodelling cycle

remodelled either to repair damage or to adapt to mechanical strain. The remodelling process follows a defined sequence where resorption precedes, and is coupled to, bone formation so that under normal circumstances the amount of bone removed is exactly balanced by that deposited (Fig. 9.4).

Resorption

The first step in resorption is the differentiation of stem cells of the monocyte–macrophage series to form committed osteoclast progenitors. These cells then fuse, probably under the major influence of $1,25(OH)_2D$, to form multi-nucleated osteoclasts which, after activation, resorb bone by removing the mineral by acid hydrolysis and then degrading the exposed collagen matrix by the secretion of proteolytic enzymes.

Once osteoclastic resorption is complete the cavity is invaded by mononuclear cells prior to the initiation of bone formation. The exact function of these mononuclear cells, probably macrophages, is uncertain. They may remove residual collagen or non-collagen proteins or they may release growth factors which stimulate osteoblast proliferation and differentiation. However, it is generally accepted that humoral factors, such as transforming growth factor β, are released during, or at the end of, resorption and are responsible for the coupling of bone resorption and formation.

Formation

Osteoblasts, derived from mesenchymal stromal cells lay down the collagen matrix which subsequently mineralizes to replace the resorbed bone. The initial phase of mineralization involves the formation of small vesicles by the osteo-blasts which migrate into the zone of mineralization. These vesicles, which are rich in alkaline phosphatase, contain small needle-like crystals of apatite whose growth depends on the uptake of calcium and phosphate from the surrounding microenvironment. Eventually the crystals grow to such a size that they rupture the vesicles and form clusters and nodules of apatite on the collagen matrix. At this stage growth of the apatite crystal is dependent on the calcium and phosphate content of the matrix rather than on the vesicles. The osteoblasts may contribute to this growth by the secretion of soluble calcium phosphate complexes which can be broken down by the alkaline phosphatase of the matrix vesicle. In the final stages of mineralization the apatite needles re-orientate in the axial direction of the collagen fibrils and form the fully calcified collagen of mature bone. This last stage will be impaired in vitamin D deficiency where there is insufficient calcium and phosphate to allow coalescence of the initial apatite deposits.

Other hormonal influences on calcium and phosphate homoeostasis

Parathyroid hormone related protein (PTHrP)

This recently isolated hormone is of particular clinical interest because it is responsible for the development of hypercalcaemia in some patients with malignancy. However, it may also have an important physiological role in the maintenance of calcium homoeostasis in the foetus and possible effects on cell differentiation in the adult.

PTHrP is a 141-amino acid peptide with biological actions similar to PTH (increased bone resorption and renal effects which include enhanced calcium reabsorption, promotion of phosphaturia and the generation of cAMP). It is at least equipotent in this respect with PTH and shows significant homology at the N-terminal region where 8 of the first 13 amino acids are identical. There-after the sequences diverge and this may explain the lack of cross-reactivity between immunoassays for these two hormones. As with PTH, the biological effects of PTHrP on bone and kidney are dependent on the 1–34 amino-terminal fragment and possibly act through the PTH receptor.

Physiological role

PTHrP can be identified histochemically in normal adult skin where it may act as a local cytokine regulating cell differentiation; hence its presence in squamous cell cancers is of particular pathophysiological interest. The source of the significant circulating levels of PTHrP in normal individuals is currently uncertain but skin seems an unlikely candidate.

PTHrP is found in epitheliae from many different sites in the human foetus but its presence in placenta and the parathyroid gland may be of particular significance. The hormone regulates placental calcium transport and may be responsible for ensuring the supply of calcium for skeletal development as well as maintaining the foetus hypercalcaemic relative to the mother. The placenta seems to be the earliest source of PTHrP although this function may be taken over by the parathyroid glands later in gestation. Regulation of placental calcium transport seems to be unique to PTHrP and this cannot be replaced by PTH or $1,25(OH)_2D$, implying that a unique receptor is involved. PTHrP is also found in maternal milk in concentrations 10 000-fold higher than plasma. Whether its role is as a local regulator of calcium transport or whether it has some effect on calcium homoeostasis in the suckling infant is uncertain.

PTHrP is also important as a humoral factor in the production of hypercalcaemia in some types of cancer, particular squamous cell tumours of the head and neck but also in those derived from kidney, breast and lymphoid tissue. The renal effects of enhanced calcium reabsorption, phosphate excretion and cAMP generation seemed to be due to PTHrP alone. The stimulatory effect on bone resorption might be a sole function of the hormone or might involve an interaction with other tumour-produced cytokines such as interleukin 1, tumour necrosis factor and transforming growth factor. Increased circulating concentrations of PTHrP in malignancy may not necessarily be associated with hypercalcaemia and this may be purely a dose-response effect or may mean that in some tumours other factors are involved.

Calcitonin

Calcitonin is a 32-amino acid peptide secreted by the parafolicular cells of the thyroid. The initial translation product is a 17 500 Da peptide containing a leader sequence which undergoes both amino- and carboxy-terminal co- and post-translational trimming to produce the secreted peptide (mol. wt. 3500). The calcitonin gene is also present in brain, where differential splicing results in the expression of calcitonin gene-related peptide (CGRP).

Calcitonin secretion is stimulated by an increase in ECF calcium and by the release of gut hormones, particularly gastrin. The physiological role of calcitonin is uncertain since patients with either very high or absent plasma concentrations seem to have no obvious abnormality of skeletal or calcium homoeostasis. Calcitonin has a transient inhibitory effect on osteoclastic bone resorption and this might give a clue to its physiological role. It has been suggested that when food arrives in the stomach, enteric hormones stimulate calcitonin release from the thyroid. This produces a transient hypocalcaemia due to an inhibition of calcium efflux from bone, which in turn will stimulate PTH release. As a consequence there will be retention by the body of the calcium absorbed from the intestine because the associated hyperparathyroidism will stimulate calcium reabsorption and thereby prevent loss of absorbed calcium in the urine. The absorbed calcium will balance the calcium retained within bone due to the action of calcitonin and ECF calcium homoeostasis will be restored.

Pharmacological doses of calcitonin are used to inhibit osteoclastic bone resorption in conditions such as Paget's disease and osteoporosis. At these levels calcitonin also inhibits calcium and sodium reabsorption by the kidney and another therapeutic use is in the promotion of calcium excretion in malignancy-associated hypercalcaemia.

CGRP has a weak calcitonin-like effect on bone but also has effects which are independent of the calcitonin receptor. CGRP acts as an arterial vasodilator, probably through release from nerve terminals innervating the vasculature and causes both a fall in blood pressure and a reflex tachycardia. The significance of these effects to normal physiology is uncertain.

Pathophysiological basis of common metabolic bone diseases

Hypercalcaemia

The common causes of hypercalcaemia and their pathophysiological basis are shown in Fig. 9.5.

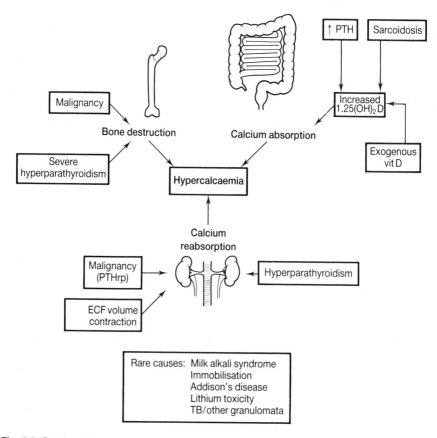

Fig. 9.5 Causes of hypercalcaemia

Hyperparathyroidism

Increased PTH secretion stimulates the renal 1α-hydroxylase to produce enhanced quantities of $1,25(OH)_2D$ which stimulates calcium and phosphate entry into the ECF from gut and bone. Excretion of the excess calcium is impaired by the stimulatory effect of PTH on distal renal tubular calcium reabsorption. The hypercalcaemia will stabilize because it will cause an increase in the filtered load of calcium (non-protein bound calcium $\times$ GFR) which will therefore increase the amount of calcium presented to the kidney for excretion. Although distal renal tubular reabsorption of calcium is enhanced, it will be relatively fixed and so an increase in filtered load will result in an increase in net calcium excretion. When this increase in calcium excretion balances the increased influx of calcium from gut and bone the serum calcium will stabilize at its new high level.

Vitamin D intoxication

Increased intake of parent vitamin D will override the weak product-inhibited hepatic 25-hydroxylase. Serum concentrations of 25-hydroxy-D will therefore rise and begin to cross-react with the intestinal and bone $1,25(OH)_2D$ receptor which has a low affinity for $25(OH)_2D$. Hence calcium influx into the ECF from bone and intestine will be stimulated. At first the increased influx of calcium into the ECF will be balanced by increased renal excretion because the tendency to hypercalcaemia will suppress PTH and inhibit distal calcium reabsorption. However, eventually the homoeostatic function of the kidney will be overwhelmed and hypercalcaemia will become established.

Overdosage by 1α-hydroxylated metabolites of vitamin D (Alfacalcidol, Calcitriol) which are used in the treatment of renal bone disease, hypoparathyroidism and vitamin D-resistant states, are potent causes of hypercalcaemia because they act directly on gut and bone as described above.

Sarcoidosis

Macrophages in the sarcoid granulomata (and in other similar granulomata) are able to convert 25-hydroxy-D into $1,25(OH)_2D$ but unlike the kidney they are unregulated by PTH or the constraints of calcium homoeostasis. Increased concentrations of $1,25(OH)_2D$ cause hypercalcaemia as described above.

Malignancy

Hypercalcaemia develops because of a number of different mechanisms. Increased bone destruction may occur either due to direct invasion of bone by malignant cells or because of stimulation of osteoclastic bone resorption by tumour products, such as PTHrP, secreted by the primary tumour or its metastases. Even if malignant cells are present in bone they may not necessarily destroy bone directly, but may secrete growth factors and cytokines into the bone microenvironment. These stimulate the normal osteoclast to resorb the trabecular surface.

The other important aspect of malignancy is the effect which occurs on the renal excretion of calcium. This is often impaired and involves a number of different mechanisms:

1. Hypercalcaemia exerts a nephrotoxic effect on the glomerulus with the result that GFR may fall, thereby limiting the ability of the kidney to excrete an unwanted calcium load. Many hypercalcaemic patients are also volume depleted (see below) and this also reduces GFR.
2. Another manifestation of the nephrotoxic effect of hypercalcaemia is the development of nephrogenic diabetes insipidus which is due to a direct effect of hypercalcaemia impairing the action of vasopressin on the collecting duct. Increased water loss (polyuria) leads to ECF volume contraction. The main defence against this is to increase the proximal renal tubular reabsorption of sodium. Unfortunately calcium reabsorption is linked to that of sodium in the proximal nephron, so ECF volume depletion further impairs the ability of the kidney to excrete unwanted calcium. These two mechanisms are common to all types of hypercalcaemia but their severity seems proportional to the height of the serum calcium particularly when values exceed 3 mmol/l.
3. Increased distal renal tubular reabsorption of calcium due to the effect of PTHrP.

Although bone resorption and formation are normally coupled they may become uncoupled in malignancy by PTHrP which seems to stimulate resorption but inhibit formation. Moreover, in malignancy there may be so much bone destruction that the bones become painful. As soon as the physical mobility of the patient becomes impaired, then gravitational stress upon which osteoblastic bone formation depends will decrease. An important consequence of this immobilization is that there will be a reduction in bone formation which 'protects' against hypercalcaemia by recycling some of the calcium from the increased resorption.

Hypocalcaemia

Hypocalcaemia is most commonly due either to a deficiency in the supply of vitamin D or PTH, or to a defect in their metabolism (Fig. 9.6; Table 9.3). As with hypercalcaemia it is the interplay between calcium fluxes between gut, bone and kidney which is involved in the development of hypocalcaemia.

Hypoparathyroidism

This may be due either to deficient secretion of PTH, usually caused by removal or damage to the glands by thyroid surgery, or to a defect in the way that PTH interacts with the receptor–adenylate cyclase complex of target cells (pseudohypoparathyroidism). This latter condition is very rare but is the classical example of an inherited hormone-resistant syndrome. PTH concentrations are high and the syndrome probably comprises a number of different defects at various stages of activation of the receptor–adenylate cyclase complex. These patients can be distinguished from those with PTH deficiency by immunoassay for intact circulating PTH or by administering exogenous PTH. This causes a 50–100-fold increase in cAMP in PTH deficiency but little response in those with PTH resistance.

PTH deficiency or resistance causes hypocalcaemia because calcium reabsorption by the distal renal tubules and efflux of calcium out of bone are decreased. In addition, the decreased activity of the PTH-stimulated 1-α-hydroxylation of 25(OH)D in the kidney results in a reduction in circulating 1,25(OH)$_2$D and a fall in calcium absorption from the gut. Plasma phosphate is raised in these patients because phosphate reabsorption is enhanced when PTH action on the kidney is deficient

Vitamin D deficiency

Hypocalcaemia is due to deficient production of 1,25(OH)$_2$D with a consequent reduction in calcium absorption from the gut and efflux out of bone.

Poor intake, or malabsorption, of vitamin D may so reduce circulating levels of 25(OH)D that 1,25(OH)$_2$D production by the kidney is reduced. Although liver disease can impair 25(OH)D production this is an unusual clinical problem because the liver has such an enormous reserve capacity. However, 25-hydroxylation of parent vitamin D may be impaired by some anticonvulsant drugs such as phenobarbitone and phenytoin. Vitamin D deficiency may also occur in biliary cirrhosis but it is the malabsorption of fat (and vitamin D) which is the central problem rather than the failure of 25-hydroxylation. Chronic renal failure will also lead to hypocalcaemia because of impaired capacity of the diseased kidney to produce 1,25(OH)$_2$D. As the supply of calcium and phosphate decreases from intestinal malabsorption there will be failure of the mineralization phase of bone remodelling leading to bone pain, deformity and a risk of fracture.

As the serum calcium level falls the parathyroid glands attempt to maintain

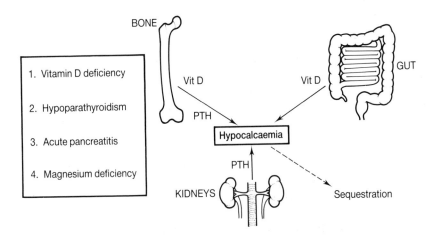

Fig. 9.6 Common causes and pathogenesis of hypocalcaemia

Table 9.3   Causes of hypocalcaemia, hypomagnesaemia and hypophosphatemia

Hypocalcaemia
  Vitamin D deficiency
  Hypoparathyroidism
  Pancreatitis

Hypomagnesaemia
  Severe diarrhoea
  Thiazide diuretics
  Alcoholism

Hypophosphataemia
  Hyperparathyroidism (primary or secondary)
  Severe diarrhoea
  Excessive use of phosphate binders, e.g. aluminium hydroxide

homoeostasis by stimulating calcium reabsorption (and phosphate excretion) by the kidney and increasing osteoclastic bone resorption. Thus the hypocalcaemia of vitamin D deficiency can be distinguished from that of hypoparathyroidism by the presence of hypophosphataemia in the former and hyperphosphataemia in the latter. In the initial stages calcium may be maintained in the lower part of the normal range but eventually the defective mineralization of bone will impair the effectiveness of osteoclastic resorption and serum calcium will fall to very low levels.

Hypomagnesaemia

Parathyroid secretion shows a biphasic response to a fall in serum magnesium. A modest fall stimulates the gland but once the serum level falls below about 0.45 mmol/l (normal 0.7 to 1 mmol/l) parathyroid hormone secretion becomes inhibited and a state of functional hypoparathyroidism occurs with effect on the calcium homoeostatic system which have already been described (Table 9.3).

Normocalcaemic disorders of bone remodelling

Osteoporosis

This is a condition where bone mineral is progressively lost so that the mechanical integrity of bone becomes impaired and fractures occur. It is due to an imbalance in the bone remodelling cycle in which there is net bone resorption. This can occur either because of an increase in bone resorption due to hypogonadism, such as occurs after the menopause in women, or at any age in men. Alternatively, bone formation may be decreased either because of the inhibitory effects of excess alcohol ingestion or by the effects of corticosteroids. The essential feature of osteoporosis is that although the degree of the uncoupling of bone turnover is only small it occurs over prolonged periods of time. The net increase in bone resorption will mean that more calcium is liberated from the bone than is deposited by formation, but since the actual amount of calcium involved is very small it can easily be excreted and does not perturb calcium homoeostasis.

Paget's disease

This is characterized by a greatly accelerated bone turnover. This seems to be due to infection of the osteoclast by a slow virus which causes the osteoclast precursors to fuse to produce giant osteoclasts. The resorbing capacity of an osteoclast is related to the number of its nuclei and so these large cells are very active. Although bone resorption may be greatly increased the coupling mechanism is preserved so that bone formation also becomes increased and bone mass is maintained. The bone architecture is abnormal, but since the amount of calcium released from the increased resorption is 'recycled' by the increased formation, no change occurs in calcium homoeostasis.

10

Hormones and the kidney

The kidneys are a pair of retroperitoneal organs which lie with their hila at an anatomical level of L1. The kidneys are highly vascularized receiving approximately 20–25 per cent (1.1 l/min) of the cardiac output via the renal arteries which are derived directly from the abdominal aorta. Each kidney consists of a medulla and surrounding cortex and under normal circumstances the cortex receives 80 per cent of the renal blood flow. At perfusion pressures between 80–180 mmHg the kidney maintains blood flow via local vasodilation and constriction of afferent and efferent blood vessels. This mechanism is termed autoregulation. The kidneys have a range of physiological functions which include:

1. Removal of nitrogenous waste products.
2. Regulation of ion status including sodium, potassium and calcium.
3. Regulation of water balance.
4. Regulation of acid-base status.
5. Hormone synthesis: endocrine and paracrine.

This chapter describes some of the hormone-sensitive facets of ion and water balance and the role of the kidney as an endocrine organ.

Ion and water balance

The functional unit of the kidney is the nephron. Each kidney contains 10^6 nephrons equivalent to a total tubule length of about 25 miles! Some 85 per cent of the nephrons lie in the cortex whilst 15 per cent span the cortico-medullary junction. This distribution of nephrons explains, at least in part, the zonal distribution of renal blood flow. Blood flows into the capillaries encircled by the Bowman's capsule of the nephron. In this capillary network the competing forces of oncotic pressure, membrane permeability and transglomerular pressure result in the plasma being 'filtered' across the glomerular basement membrane. When the plasma filtrate lies in the lumen of nephron it is referred to as the glomerular filtrate (GF). Approximately 170 litres of GF are produced each day but only 1–2 litres of urine are ultimately produced. Clearly an efficient mechanism for the absorption of water and solutes from the initial GF must exist and it is the regulation of these processes which allow ion and water homoeostasis to be achieved. The initial glomerular filtrate has a composition which is very similar to that of plasma. In fact the only major difference between plasma and GF is that the larger serum proteins have been excluded from the GF by virtue of the permeability barrier created by the glomerular basement membrane (ultrafiltration). Some small molecular weight proteins do pass into the glomerular filtrate but these and molecules such as glucose are usually completely reabsorbed as the filtrate passes down the nephron. The presence of protein or glucose in the urine may have pathological implications (see Chapter 6, Diabetes mellitus).

Ions

The concentration of all ions found in the serum is regulated by the balance of supply (diet, etc.), absorption (GI tract, skin), distribution (storage and mobilization of stores, e.g. in adipose tissue and liver) and excretion (renal and faecal). Ions in plasma pass unhindered into the glomerular filtrate and so the regulation of excretion rate is achieved by modulating the rate of ion reabsorption (or active secretion) as the filtrate passes down the length of the nephron. Reabsorption is affected by a number of factors which include:

1. The rate of glomerular filtration, filtrate passage time and filtrate volume.
2. Carrier-mediated, specific, active transport mechanisms (ATP-dependent).
3. Passive diffusion along ion concentration gradients.
4. Passive diffusion along electrochemical gradients.

The bulk of the reabsorption activity (up to 75 per cent) takes place in the proximal tubule and is not usually subject to hormonal regulation. In the distal tubule, however, the 'fine tuning' of ion excretion is subject to hormonal control.

Sodium and water homoeostasis

The regulation of serum sodium concentration and total body water content are intimately interconnected, but for the sake of simplicity will be discussed separately here.

Sodium

The fluid content of an average 70 kg man is about 42 litres (60 per cent of body weight) and is distributed across a number of physiological/anatomical 'compartments'. Some 60 per cent (28 litres) of the water is intracellular plasma whilst the remaining 30 per cent (14 litres) is present in the extracellular compartment (interstitial fluid). Although water is freely mobile between these compartments ions are not, and the distribution of water between these 'compartments' is therefore governed by forces which operate across all semi-permeable membranes which include: osmotic gradients (created by solutes such as glucose, sodium and potassium); oncotic gradients (reflecting protein concentrations); hydrostatic pressure (blood pressure, peripheral vascular resistance and venous pressure); membrane permeability and surface area. Consideration of these factors gives considerable insight into the conditions which can give rise to expansion of the extravascular fluid volume and result in oedema (peripheral oedema and pleural, peritoneal and pericardial effusions). Reduced oncotic pressure (due to protein loss, e.g. nephrotic syndrome or GI disease), increased hydrostatic pressure (e.g. in right-sided heart failure) and increased membrane permeability (e.g. inflammation secondary to infection or neoplasia) can all result in a shift of fluid from the vascular or intracellular compartments to the extracellular (and extravascular) space. Changes in plasma osmotic pressure can also cause fluid shifts. An approximate value of the osmotic potential of extracellular fluid may be calculated from the equation:

$$2(Na^+ + K^+) + glucose + urea = 275\text{--}295 \text{ mOsmol}$$

Sodium, at a plasma concentration of 135–142 mmol/l, is the most abundant extracellular cation and is the single most important factor in determining plasma osmolarity. Sodium clearly plays an essential role in the regulation of plasma volume and it is therefore not surprising that the plasma volume is a major regulatory influence on the total body content of sodium. Increases in total body sodium lead to expansion of the extracellular and vascular fluid space whilst sodium depletion can cause a decline in extracellular and vascular volume which if extreme enough can compromise the cardiovascular system, leading to hypovolaemic circulatory failure. Five major but inter-related mechanisms exist to control the rate of sodium excretion (and regulate plasma volume). These are listed and discussed below:

1. Distribution of renal blood flow.
2. Peritubular reabsorption pressure.
3. Renin, angiotensin and aldosterone.
4. Cortisol–cortisone shuttle.
5. Natriuretic factor.

Distribution of renal blood flow

Under normal conditions renal blood flow is directed predominantly to the cortex where a majority of the nephrons are located. However, it is the cortical–medullary nephrons which have the highest capacity for sodium reabsorption. Under conditions where sodium conservation is required, local, possibly prostaglandin-mediated, vasoactive mechanisms act to redistribute the renal flow to the cortico–medullary nephrons, thereby increasing the capacity for sodium reabsorption.

Peritubular reabsorption pressure

Changes in the rate of renal blood flow can cause alterations in the composition of the peritubular fluid with consequences for water and ion movements. Reduced renal blood flow increases the transit time of blood through the Bowman's capsule, allowing more fluid to move across the basement membrane. This results in a relative increase in the protein concentration of the peritubular fluid, increasing the transluminal oncotic pressure. These conditions favour the movement of water (and ions) from the renal tubule into the peritubular fluid.

Such a mechanism would increase sodium retention in situations of reduced renal blood flow which are interpreted by the kidney as reflecting situations of low plasma volume and sodium depletion.

Renin, angiotensin and aldosterone

Aldosterone is a mineralocorticosteroid produced in the zona glomerulosa of the adrenal cortex. Its principal action is to promote sodium reabsorption and potassium excretion in the distal tubule of the nephron, although it also affects sodium transport and distribution in other body fluids, e.g. saliva. Only 10 per cent of the initial tubular sodium load reaches the distal tubule and it has been calculated that only 20 per cent of this (i.e. 2 per cent of the total sodium load) is sensitive to the effects of aldosterone. Although this appears to be a very small proportion of the total sodium load, it can be calculated that aldosterone potentially prevents the loss of 504 mmol of sodium per day (GFR: (180 l/d) $\times$ Na^+ (140 mM) $\times$ 2 per cent), which is equivalent to 30 g of table salt.

Aldosterone appears to have both acute and chronic effects on sodium reabsorption. The acute effects are probably mediated by activation of pre-existing sodium channels. This activation appears to be energy dependent and possibly involves aldosterone-mediated methylation of, or Ca^{2+} binding to, the sodium channel protein. The exact mechanisms mediating the acute effects of aldosterone are unknown. The more chronic effects of aldosterone are seen 45–90 minutes after exposure to aldosterone and as with other steroid hormones require the binding of aldosterone to cytosolic receptors present in the target cells. The receptor–hormone complex enters the nucleus where it binds to DNA-binding proteins initiating the transcription of specific genes into mRNA. The mRNA is translocated into the cytoplasm and translated into specific proteins which mediate the cellular response to the hormone. Aldosterone stimulates the synthesis of specific proteins which increase luminal membrane permeability to sodium, mitochondrial ATP production and Na^+/K^+ ATPase activity.

The secretion of aldosterone from the zona glomerulosa of the adrenal cortex is stimulated by a number of different factors:(i) adrenocorticotrophic hormone (ACTH); (ii) plasma sodium and potassium; (iii) renin-angiotensin system.

ACTH

ACTH is a peptide hormone produced by the anterior pituitary gland. Its major function is to stimulate the adrenal cortex to produce the glucocorticoid hormone, cortisol. At high concentrations ACTH stimulates aldosterone production but it is generally felt that this effect is of minor physiological significance.

Sodium and potassium concentrations

Aldosterone secretion is stimulated by a rise in serum potassium or a fall in serum sodium concentrations. Although of some importance this is not the main regulator of aldosterone secretion.

Renin and angiotensin system (RAS)

The RAS constitutes the major regulator of aldosterone release (Fig 10.1). The mRNA for renin has been found in a number of tissues including brain, adrenal gland, uterus and placenta. It is, however, generally agreed that the kidney is the physiologically most important site of renin synthesis. This assertion is supported by the observations that serum renin concentrations fall significantly following bilateral nephrectomy. In the kidney renin is synthesized and stored as a preprohormone in cells of the juxtaglomerular complex. Renin release is stimulated by a number of factors which are influenced by changes in sodium

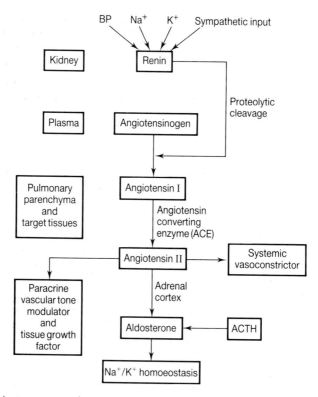

Fig. 10.1 Aldosterone cascade

load and plasma volume and include reduced sodium intake, decreased arterial pressure, a fall in extracellular fluid volume, stress and trauma. These effectors influence renin release via three basic mechanisms:

1. Local macula densa cell events. The macula cells detect the sodium content of the tubular fluid emerging from the ascending limb of the loop of Henle and communicate this information to the juxtaglomerular complex. A fall in sodium load stimulates renin release, whilst excessive sodium loads result in a fall in renin secretion.
2. Baroreceptor-mediated events. Renin secretion is modulated by renal perfusion pressure which is detected by baroreceptors located in juxtaglomerular cells or associated endothelial cells. A fall in perfusion pressure, possibly reflecting a reduction in extracellular fluid volume, stimulates renin secretion.
3. Modulation of sympathetic outflow. The juxtaglomerular cells are heavily innervated with sympathetic neurones. Low intensity β-sympathetic stimulation increases, and α-sympathetic stimulation reduces, renin secretion. High intensity sympathetic activity stimulates renin secretion directly as well as promoting an indirect release of renin via changes in haemodynamic status.

The cellular second messenger signalling mechanisms by which these various effectors modulate renin release are currently under investigation. It has been shown that the signals from macula cells and baroreceptors induce a fall in the cytosolic Ca^{2+} concentration of the juxtaglomerular cells. Other effectors of renin release appear to activate adenylate cyclase but it remains unclear if this represents a signalling system which is completely distinct from the well described Ca^{2+}-mediated mechanisms. Stimulation of renin secretion initiates the breakdown of the prohormone to an active glycoprotein with a molecular weight of 36 000–42 000 kDa. Renin appears to circulate in the serum in active and inactive forms (indeed the amount of inactive renin exceeds that of the active protease) and it has been suggested that the inactive enzyme represents prorenin which has not been activated during secretion. Active renin is an aspartyl protease which acts specifically on the substrate angiotensinogen.

Angiotensinogen is a glycoprotein (Mol.wt 52 000–60 000 kDa) which circulates in the α-globulin fraction of plasma proteins. Cleavage of angiotensinogen produces a decapeptide angiotensin I, which is itself a substrate for angiotensin-converting enzyme (ACE). ACE is a non-specific dipeptidylcarboxy-peptidase which acts on a variety of peptides including bradykinin and angiotensin I. ACE acts on angiotensin I to produce the active hormone angiotensin II. In addition, ACE inactivates the vasodilator bradykinin (see below). A major site of ACE activity is the lung parenchyma and activation of circulating angiotensin I occurs as blood passes through the pulmonary circulation. However, the importance of systemically-generated angiotensin II has been questioned. It is well known that angiotensin II has a very short plasma half-life (in the order of 1–2 minutes) and it has been estimated that 90 per cent of systemically-delivered angiotensin II is destroyed in a single pass through the kidney. The observation that ACE is present in a variety of tissue sites has given rise to the concept that the angiotensin II may be generated at its site of action and act as a paracrine hormone. In the adrenal cortex angiotensin II acts as an activator of aldosterone secretion, with subsequent sodium retention and expansion of the extracellular volume. Angiotensin II also modulates systemic vascular resistance, systemic blood pressure and local blood flow via its action as a powerful vasoconstrictor.

Angiotensin II is rapidly converted to angiotensin III by the enzyme angiotensinase. The pressor activity of angiotensin III is only 20–30 per cent that of angiotensin II; however, the two are equally potent stimulators of aldosterone secretion. The exact physiological role of angiotensin III is unknown. In rats, similar concentrations of angiotensin II and III are found in the plasma, suggesting it may have an important role. In man only a small amount of angiotensin III can be detected in the circulation however, the presence in the adrenal cortex of an aminopeptidase which converts angiotensin II to angiotensin III suggests that angiotensin III may have a physiological role in the stimulation of aldosterone release. Both angiotensin II and III activate aldosterone secretion via the inositol 1,4,5-trifphosphate/Ca^{2+} second messenger system (see Chapter 1).

In addition to modulating aldosterone secretion angiotensin II is a powerful vasoconstrictor, increasing peripheral vascular resistance and systemic blood pressure. These effects on systemic blood pressure are reinforced by the inhibitory activity of ACE on the vasodilatory kinin, bradykinin. The pressor activity of angiotensin II may be modulated, at least in part, by the opposing action of the vasodilatory prostaglandins PGI_2 and PGE_2. Angiotensin II is a powerful stimulant of PGI_2 and PGE_2 synthesis and release of these prostaglandins would temper the vasopressor activity of angiotensin II.

Angiotensin II also acts as a powerful CNS thirst stimulant. This also has implications for the regulation of plasma volume and osmolarity and will be discussed later in connection with water homoeostasis.

More recently interest has been generated in the role of locally-generated angiotensin II as a local vascular tone modulator and a paracrine growth factor. This may have particular importance in the understanding of hypertension, hypertension-related left ventricular hypertrophy, and arterial intimal thickening.

Cortisol/cortisone shuttle

Recently it has become apparent that the kidney distal tubule displays a novel, if not unique, biochemical mechanism by which the activity of the mineralocorticoid receptor responsible for sodium reabsorption is regulated. As already discussed, the major endocrine regulator of sodium reabsorption is aldosterone which binds to a mineralocorticoid receptor in the distal tubule. *In vitro* this receptor also has a high affinity for cortisol which *in vivo* is present at a concentration 100-fold greater than that of aldosterone. These observations made it difficult to explain the apparent specificity of this receptor for aldosterone *in vivo*. However, the study of the rare clinical syndrome of apparent mineralocorticoid excess (11β-hydroxysteroid dehydrogenase deficiency) and the drug glycyrrhizic acid (a 11β-hydroxysteroid dehyrodrogenase inhibitor) have shown that the specificity of the mineralocorticoid receptor for aldosterone is conferred by the activity of the enzyme 11β-hydroxysteroid dehydrogenase. It is suggested that this enzyme, which is in close association with or in fact part of, the mineralocorticoid receptor, protects the ligand binding site from cortisol by 'shuttling' active cortisol to inactive corticosterone. The consequences of unrestricted cortisol binding are seen in the syndrome of apparent mineralocorticoid excess where the 11β-hydroxysteroid deficiency leads to cortisol activation of the mineralocorticoid receptor with sodium retention, potassium loss (hypokalaemia) and hypertension. Similarly the inhibition of the enzyme with glycyrrhizic acid produces sodium retention and hypertension. It has been suggested that a partial enzyme deficiency may explain some 25 per cent of currently-labelled essential hypertension. Studies into the molecular genetics of such a defect are presently being performed.

Natriuretic factor

Natriuretic factor comprises the only system so far identified which actually promotes sodium excretion. The existence of a natriuretic hormone had been proposed, on theoretical grounds, for many years but at the time of the last edition of this text it remained a 'hypothetical' hormone. Since that time natriuretic factor has been identified and many of its biochemical and physiological functions have been determined. Atrial natriuretic peptide (ANP) is synthesized in the myocytes of the right atrium and ventricle. In rats the hormone has been shown to be synthesized as a pre-prohormone of 152 amino acids. Cleavage of this molecule produces a prohormone of 126 amino acids. The active peptide is secreted as a 28-amino acid peptide with a 17-amino acid ring structure. In common with a number of peptide hormones it circulates in the plasma in an unbound form. Pharmacological studies have suggested that ANP binds to two separate receptors. The B-receptor appears to mediate a majority of ANP's functions via a G-protein-linked guanine cyclase mechanism. A C-receptor has also been identified, which appears to stimulate the formation of inositol 1,4,5-triphosphate (IP_3), but the physiological significance of this observation is unknown. It has been suggested that the C-receptor may mediate ANP clearance.

ANP secretion appears to be stimulated by conditions which exert stress and tension of the myocytes in the right atrium and ventricle of the heart. These conditions include states which increase preload (e.g. fluid overload and sodium retention) and afterload (e.g. in hypertension and conditions which increase peripheral vascular resistance). ANP inhibits reabsorption and promotes excretion of sodium by direct and indirect mechanisms. ANP appears to act directly on the kidney by reducing the rate of tubular sodium reabsorption. In addition, ANP is a powerful local vasodilator and can reduce sodium reabsorption via haemodynamic effects on interstitial osmotic pressure and glomerular filtration. ANP also interacts with other hormone systems which act on sodium and water homoeostasis. ANP inhibits renin secretion by direct effects on the juxtaglomerular complex and reduces the rate of basal and stimulated aldosterone production by the adrenal cortex. Such actions serve to reduce sodium reabsorption and reduce vascular tone, which in turn reduces cardiac work load and myocyte stretching, thereby providing a negative feedback control loop for ANP secretion.

ANP also appears to have CNS effects which include a reduction in salt-seeking feeding behaviour and a reduction in thirst response which is probably mediated by a direct inhibitory effect of ANP on vasopressin (ADH) release (see below). More recently it has been reported that ANP stimulates growth hormone release but the physiological significance of this observation is as yet unknown.

Integration of control of sodium excretion

The regulation of sodium excretion is, in essence, the regulation of plasma volume as illustrated by factors which stimulate renin release, e.g. reduced renal perfusion pressure, adrenergic outflow, reduced tubular sodium, extracellular fluid volume and stress. A fall in blood pressure would stimulate adrenergic drive, inducing peripheral vasoconstriction in an attempt to maintain systemic blood pressure. Increased sympathetic drive and any fall in renal perfusion would in turn stimulate sodium reabsorption and expansion in plasma volume. These effects would be mediated by alterations in tubular pressure and sodium concentration, distribution of renal blood flow and stimulation of aldosterone secretion. Angiotensin II would also increase peripheral vasoconstriction, assisting in the maintenance of systemic blood pressure. In addition, the paracrine effects of angiotensin II and prostaglandins PGI_2 and PGE_2 synthesis on vascular tone would regulate local patterns of blood flow, allowing the maintenance of blood supply to specific organs. Angiotensin II may also stimulate thirst centres and salt-directed eating behaviour. Conversely, expansion of the plasma volume results in stretching of the myocardium and secretion of ANP which results in a marked excretion of sodium (natriuresis). Renin secretion would also be inhibited, and vascular tone decreased, due to a fall in serum angiotensin II levels and reduced adrenergic activity. These mechanisms are shown in Fig. 10.2.

Clinical aspects

The problems related to disorders of salt balance are principally related to fluid overload and systemic hypertension.

Hyperaldosteronism (excess aldosterone secretion) may occur as a primary or secondary disorder. Primary hyperaldosteronism (Conn's syndrome) is the autonomous production of aldosterone by an adrenal adenoma (or following bilateral adrenal hyperplasia or nodular hyperplasia). An uncontrolled increase in aldosterone production results in hypernatraemia, hypokalaemia, a mild metabolic alkalosis and hypertension. Treatment with the aldosterone antagonist, spironolactone, can reverse these changes. In contrast, aldosterone deficiency, as seen in Addison's disease (isolated aldosterone deficiency or resistance is rare) results in hyponatraemia, hyperkalaemia, a metabolic acidosis, profound hypovolaemia and hypotension.

Secondary hyperaldosteronism occurs in liver and cardiac failure. In liver failure the hyperaldosteronism results from a combination of reduced hepatic

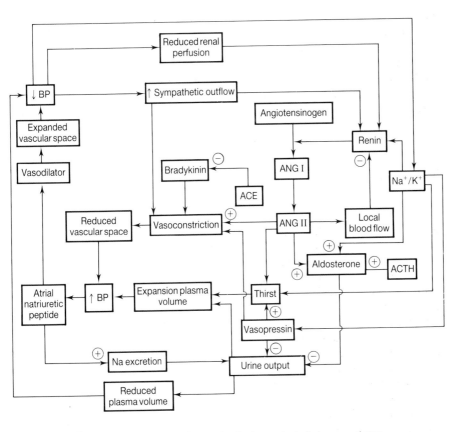

Fig. 10.2 Hormonal and neurological interaction in the control of plasma volume

aldosterone metabolism and reduced renal perfusion as a consequence of blood shunting to the peripheries. Cardiac failure is an example of a physiological regulatory mechanism being activated inappropriately with pathological consequences. Declining cardiac function (as a result of cardiac damage) results in a fall in systemic blood pressure and renal perfusion pressure. These signals are interpreted as indicating fluid/salt depletion and a number of powerful mechanisms are activated to increase sodium retention, extracellular fluid volume expansion and vasopressor activity. However, in cardiac failure these 'physiological' events are inappropriate and actually result in a worsening of cardiac function. Increased fluid load (increasing cardiac preload) stretches and dilates the heart, eventually reducing cardiac efficiency (Starling's Law, consult any physiology text). In addition, increased pressor activity elevates peripheral vascular resistance (cardiac afterload). The combined effects of an increased cardiac pre- and afterload put increased stress on an already compromised heart, resulting in a decline in cardiac output and renal perfusion. Clearly a vicious cycle has been created which if unchecked will lead to death through heart failure (inability to increase cardiac output to supply basic physiological needs). Treatment is directed at reducing peripheral vascular resistance by inhibiting

ACE (using angiotensin converting enzyme inhibitors), lowering angiotensin II levels and increasing salt and fluid excretion (using diuretics).

Potassium

Potassium is predominantly an intracellular ion and plasma concentrations are a very poor indicator of total body potassium levels. The systems regulating potassium homoeostasis are still poorly understood but appear to be partially hormone-dependent and in part related to the concentration and excretion of other ions, in particular H^+. As in the case of sodium, most of the potassium reabsorption takes place in the proximal tubule under the influence of ion and electrochemical gradients. It has been suggested that the hypokalaemia induced by diuretics is due to reduced rates of proximal tubular reabsorption. Approximately 10 per cent of the total potassium load reaches the distal tubule where both reabsorption and excretion occur. The regulation of the urinary potassium excretion rate is achieved by the balance of these opposing processes. Potassium excretion is influenced by aldosterone (aldosterone secretion is directly stimulated by hypokalaemia) which stimulates sodium retention and potassium secretion (see above). Disorders of aldosterone secretion are associated with potassium (and hydrogen ion) abnormalities. Excessive aldosterone production (Conn's syndrome) is associated with hypokalaemia and an alkalosis, while aldosterone deficiency (e.g. Hypoadrenalism disease) is characterized by hyperkalaemia and a mild metabolic acidosis. Potassium transport across the renal tubular (and cell) membrane is closely and competitively linked to hydrogen ion (H^+) excretion. In metabolic acidosis where the hydrogen ion load is increased potassium excretion is reduced. Conversely, in metabolic alkalosis where the hydrogen ion load is decreased there is an increase in urinary potassium loss. This is particularly evident in hyperemesis where loss of H^+ in the vomitus creates a metabolic alkalosis. This results in a marked increase in urinary potassium excretion and a systemic hypokalaemia.

Calcium

The kidney has a vital role in the maintenance of calcium homoeostasis both directly by regulation of calcium excretion via the action of parathyroid hormone on the distal renal tubule and indirectly through the synthesis of $1,25(OH)D_3$ via the action of the renal 1α-hydroxylase enzyme on $25(OH)D_2$. Active vitamin D influences Ca^{2+} absorption from the gut and deposition of Ca^{2+} in the skeleton. This is discussed more fully in Chapter 9.

Regulation of water content

As previously discussed the regulation of body water is intimately linked with that of body sodium. However, in contrast to sodium homoeostasis where the major regulator appears to be plasma volume, water homoeostasis appears to be primarily governed by plasma osmolarity. As with all dynamic states the steady state represents a balance between input and output, in this case fluid intake (water: fluid and food) and fluid output (urine, sweat, faeces and expired air). The major sites of regulation appear to be the control of urinary volume and regulation of fluid (and salt) intake.

Urinary output

Less than 10 per cent of the initial glomerular filtrate reaches the distal tubule. The osmolarity of the fluid in the distal tubule is approximately 150 mOsmolar, i.e. hypotonic with respect to plasma, and reflects the increased secretion of water (with respect to solute) into the tubule which occurs during the passage of the filtrate through the ascending loop of Henle. It is the reabsorption of water present in the distal tubule which is subject to regulation by antidiuretic hormone (ADH).

Antidiuretic hormone (vasopressin) is an octapeptide synthesized in the neurones of the supraoptic hypothalamic nuclei. It is bound to a protein (neurophysin II) and transported by axonal flow to the terminal bulbs of the neurones in the posterior pituitary. Release of the hormone from the posterior pituitary is stimulated by an increase in the osmolarity of blood perfusing the hypothalamus (direct stimulation of osmoreceptors) and inhibited by an increase in plasma volume, detected by baroreceptors in the left atrium. ADH acts primarily on the distal tubule, increasing tubular permeability. It binds to specific receptors on the tubular membrane and increases intracellular cAMP concentration by activating adenylate cyclase. Tubular permeability is increased via dilation of membrane pores. There is some evidence to suggest that prolonged ADH stimulation can also cause an increase in the number of functional pores. Water moves passively in accord with the existing osmotic gradient. The osmolarity of tubular fluid/urine may be raised to 1000 mOsmolar under the influence of ADH.

In addition to these actions ADH also has a minor vasoactive role, causing vasoconstriction of arteriolar and capillary beds. One consequence of this vasoconstriction would be a fall in renal blood flow. Decreased renal blood flow with a constant GFR results in increased water reabsorption in the proximal tubules. In addition these factors will stimulate the renin–angiotensin system, promoting salt and fluid retention.

Osmolarity can also be influenced by water intake. Decreased plasma volume, usually associated with an increased plasma osmolarity, serves as a direct and powerful stimulatory effect on the CNS thirst centre. In addition angiotensin II produced in response to a reduced plasma volume can act as a thirst centre stimulant and initiate salt-seeking feeding behaviour.

Clinical aspects

Diabetes insipidus (DI), has two distinct aetiologies:

1. Cranial diabetes insipidus, where decreased production of ADH by the posterior pituitary occurs as a result of surgery, carcinoma or trauma.
2. Nephrogenic diabetes insipidus; this is an inborn error in which the renal tubules are insensitive to ADH.

In DI, the hormone ADH is either deficient or ineffective and the ability of the kidney to concentrate urine becomes severely impaired. Patients therefore produce large volumes of dilute urine and drink large quantities of fluid. The ensuing prolonged diuresis leads to dehydration, hypotension and a state of hypernatraemia. Even under extreme conditions, e.g. maintained fluid loss but with severe fluid intake restriction, the kidneys remain unable to concentrate the urine and conserve water. This observation forms the basis of the water deprivation test which is used to differentiate between patients with DI and psychogenic polydipsia.

In nephrogenic diabetes insipidus drugs which augment the action of ADH (chloropropamide, carbamazepine) may be useful. However, synthetic ADH is available (DDAVP) as a snuff and this can ameliorate both forms of diabetes insipidus.

ADH secretion can be inhibited by a number of drugs, including alcohol. The inhibitory effect of alcohol on posterior pituitary function (it also inhibits oxytocin and was in the past used to slow uterine contractions in premature labour) may explain the diuresis which accompanies alcohol consumption.

Syndromes of inappropriate ADH secretion are also recognized and these are characterized by the presence of hyponatraemia in a patient who clinically has normal fluid balance (e.g. not sodium depleted or fluid overloaded). This condition occurs as a consequence of a variety of intracranial and chest disorders including carcinoma of the lung. Treatment by water restriction usually ameliorates the condition although occasionally drugs of the tetracycline group, e.g. desmocycline, which inhibit the tubular activity of ADH, are used.

Other hormones and renal function

A number of hormones have been shown to exert effects on the kidney tubule: these include glucagon, parathyroid hormone, calcitonin and epidermal growth factor. All appear to stimulate adenylate cyclase activity in specific areas of the nephron. Glucagon, PTH and calcitonin appear to act on the thick ascending limb (TAL) of the loop of Henle and to be involved in water conservation, though the exact physiological significance of these observations is unknown (the effects of PTH on Ca^{2+} and Mg^{2+} are discussed elsewhere). Epidermal growth factor (EGF, a 53-amino acid peptide) is produced in the TAL and it has been suggested that it may act as a paracrine regulator of tubular function. In sheep EGF induces a diuresis and natriuresis and strongly inhibits vasopressin action in the cortical collecting ducts.

Acid–base metabolism

The regulation of the acid–base status involves the interaction of both the respiratory and renal systems. The most important reaction in understanding acid–base regulation is:

$$CO_2 + H_2O = H_2CO_3 \gtrless H^+ + HCO^-_3$$

The synthesis of carbonic acid (H_2CO_3) is catalysed by the zinc-dependent enzyme carbonic anhydrase which is present in erythrocytes and renal tubular cells. The dissociation of carbonic acid to bicarbonate and hydrogen ion is dependent on the prevailing concentrations of these ions in the tissue/plasma/renal tubule. The production and disposal of CO_2 is quantitatively the most important determinant of overall acid–base status and under normal circumstances a majority of the acid produced by processes such as metabolic oxidation is disposed of as CO_2 via the lungs (volatile acids). The remaining H^+ ions produced from activities such as ketogenesis and lactic acid formation are either buffered or excreted by the distal tubule as ammonium or hydrogen phosphate ions with the net synthesis of bicarbonate. Pathological states which affect renal or respiratory function or influence the production of metabolic acids can lead to alterations in the acid–base status (respiratory or metabolic acidosis or alkalosis).

Respiratory influences

The respiratory system contributes to the acid–base status by influencing the level of CO_2 in the blood. Ventilation is the most important regulator of blood CO_2 levels; hyperventilation (e.g. anxiety) removes CO_2 creating a respiratory alkalosis whilst hypoventilation (e.g. brain injury, drug overdose) leads to CO_2 accumulation and a respiratory acidosis. The H^+ concentration of the CSF, which reflects plasma pH, is a powerful regulator of ventilation rate and so metabolically-induced acid–base disturbances can be compensated for by changes in ventilation rate. A metabolic acidosis (e.g. diabetic ketoacidosis or renal failure) will stimulate an increase in respiratory rate, lowering CO_2 and correcting the metabolic acidosis by inducing a respiratory alkalosis. Similarly a metabolic alkalosis will result in hypoventilation with consequent accumulation of CO_2 and a compensatory respiratory alkalosis.

Renal influences

The metabolic compensation for respiratory-induced alterations in acid–base status are easy to understand if the reaction of carbonic anhydrase is consulted (see above). An increase in CO_2 (respiratory acidosis due to hypoventilation) will result in the displacement of the reaction to the right with the subsequent excretion of H^+ and synthesis of bicarbonate. This net acid excretion and regeneration of bicarbonate leads to a correction of the respiratory acidosis. Conversely, a respiratory alkalosis will lead to a reduced rate of acid secretion and bicarbonate generation and the creation of a compensatory metabolic acidosis.

Under normal circumstances all filtered bicarbonate is reabsorbed in the proximal tubule. This process is increased in the presence of a high pCO_2 (emphasizing the importance of CO_2 in acid–base metabolism and the inter-relation of respiratory and renal systems) hypernatraemia and hypokalaemia. Distal tubular acid secretion is associated with sodium reabsorption and this explains the observation that the ability to cope with an acid load is dependent on salt status.

If acid production exceeds the capacity of these mechanisms to compensate bicarbonate depletion, H^+ accumulation leads to the development of a metabolic acidosis. Metabolic acidoses have been classified into type A and type B. Type A is the most common clinical situation and is defined as a metabolic acidosis in the presence of hypotension and hypoxia. Type B is more unusual and is usually precipitated by drugs (metformin, phenformin and alcohol) particularly in patients with hepatic and renal disease.

Once a metabolic acidosis has developed, respiratory mechanisms (hyperventilation: see above) attempt to compensate. If this compensation is unsuccessful a self-perpetuating cycle can develop and this situation is exemplified by diabetic ketoacidosis (DKA). In DKA increased ketogenesis (due to insulin deficiency; see Chapter 6) leads to an increased renal H^+ load. The diuresis induced by hyperglycaemia results in dehydration, hypovolaemia and sodium depletion, all of which impair bicarbonate reabsorption and acid excretion and exacerbate the acidosis. The increasing acidosis further impairs renal function and also diminishes myocardial efficiency. Impaired cardiac output (hypovolaemia and myocardial depression) reduces peripheral tissue perfusion, inducing tissue hypoxia and promoting lactic acid production which further perpetuates the metabolic acidosis.

In clinical practice infusion of intravenous saline (salt and fluid replacement: reversing the hypovolaemia and improving renal acid handling) and insulin (inhibiting ketone synthesis) can improve renal function to a level where acid–base homoeostasis can be re-established (see Chapter 6; Diabetes mellitus).

Erythropoietin

The presence of a renally-derived growth factor which controls red cell synthesis (erythrogenesis) has been known since 1957. It is now known that the kidney is the major site of synthesis of the hormone erythropoietin (EP) which is a powerful and specific erythroid growth factor. A small amount of EP synthesis takes place in the liver but other than during foetal life this extrarenal source probably has limited physiological significance. Over recent years EP has been purified, sequenced and cloned and a human recombinant EP is now in clinical use. The intrarenal site of EP synthesis is currently unknown but appears to be in cells associated with the proximal renal tubules. EP synthesis is principally controlled by the serum O_2 tension. Hypoxia is a powerful stimulant to EP production with a resultant increase in red cell mass and O_2-carrying potential. The mechanism by which O_2 tension is detected in the renal tubule is currently unknown but possibly involves a haem-containing receptor protein. The second messenger controlling EP synthesis is also unknown but candidates include cyclic AMP and reduced cytoplasmic Ca^{2+}. In addition to hypoxia androgens, cobalt ions and PGE_2 also stimulate EP synthesis (Fig. 10.3). The effect of androgens explains why men have higher haematocrits than women and why androgens have been used in the treatment of aplastic anaemia. It is of some interest that stimulation of EP synthesis appears to result in an increased number of cells producing EP rather than simply increasing the rate of EP synthesis in cells already producing the hormone.

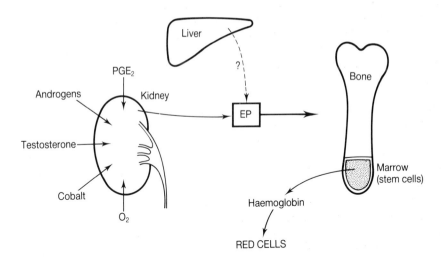

Fig. 10.3 Erythropoeitin production

Considerable data exist concerning the structure and molecular biology of EP and the EP receptor. This will be discussed briefly.

EP structure and molecular biology

The gene for EP is on chromosome 7 in man and 5 in the mouse. The gene is present as a single copy and is 7 kb pairs long and composed of 4-introns and 5-exons. The gene codes for a peptide which is 193 peptides long. A 27-amino acid leader sequence is cleaved from the prohormone on secretion, producing a 166-amino acid peptide (mol. wt. 18 397 Da). However, the bioactive hormone is heavily glycosylated (30–40 per cent), bringing the molecular weight to 34 000 Da.

EP receptor

The gene for the EP receptor is on chromosome 19. The EP receptor has structural similarities to the receptors for IL-2,-3,-6,-7, GM-CSF, G-CSF, prolactin and growth hormone. All these receptors appear to have a cytokine binding domain and it has been suggested that they constitute a haemopoietin receptor 'super family'. Despite all this detailed information the second messenger for the EP receptor remains unknown.

Clinical aspects

The availability of recombinant human erythropoietin has been a major therapeutic advance. The most obvious (and successful) application has been in patients with chronic renal failure who cannot produce EP and consequently suffer from a profound and debilitating anaemia. Treatment with EP can normalize the red cell mass in these patients with a dramatic improvement in their quality of life. Several therapeutic problems have become apparent and these include the development of severe hypertension and an increased tendency to undergo spontaneous thrombotic events. These complications are now actively screened for and treatment monitored and adjusted accordingly.

The dramatic improvements in sporting performance which accompany altitude training have been attributed to the increased red cell mass induced by hypoxia (and EP secretion). Inevitably therefore EP has found its way into the 'sports drug scene'. EP has been nicknamed 'go-juice' and is apparently being taken by large numbers of endurance athletes, particularly cyclists. Unfortunately these athletes do not have the benefit of medical supervision and the complications from EP therapy, previously noted, go undetected. It has been suggested that the recent spate of deaths in young competitive cyclists, apparently from myocardial infarction, may be due to coronary thrombosis occurring as a consequence of EP-induced polycythaemia.

Ectopic and inappropriate EP production is well recognized clinically and the polycythaemia associated with renal cell carcinoma and phaeochromocytomas has been shown to be the result of ectopic EP production.

Prostaglandin synthesis

Recent evidence suggests that the kidney is a very active site of prostaglandin synthesis, especially PGI_2 and PGE_2. These compounds are powerful vasodilators and can effect dramatic changes in local blood flow and reductions in systemic blood pressure. Recent interest in these compounds has been generated by the observation that insulin and corticosteroids inhibit the production of these prostaglandins whilst angiotensin II and ADH stimulate their synthesis and release. These prostaglandins may also have a role in the regulation of renin secretion and water excretion (independent of ADH). The clinical implications of these observations in conditions such as essential hypertension and hypertension associated with diabetes mellitus is currently being reviewed.

Kallikrenin–kinin system

The kinins are a group of paracrine peptides which are produced in a number of sites including the kidney. Kinins are produced via proteolytic activation of inactive kallikrenins in a system analogous to the RAS. Indeed, the two systems are interconnected by virtue of ACE, which activates angiotensin I and inhibits bradykinin. In the kidney kallikrenin, a peptidase produced in the renal cortex, acts on kininogen, releasing an active molecule, bradykinin. Bradykinin is a powerful vasodilator and may be involved in the regulation of renal blood flow. There is some evidence to suggest that the kinin system may also be involved in sodium homoeostasis (bradykinin can induce natriuresis) but its physiological role in these processes is as yet undefined.

Bradykinin activates the enzyme phospholipase A_2 which acts on phospholipids to produce arachidonic acid, a precursor for prostaglandin synthesis (e.g. PGE_2 and PGI_2). As already discussed these agents are powerful vasodilators and may compliment the action of bradykinin. In addition, PGE_2 and PGI_2

are also implicated in the control cycle of the RAS that also impinges on the kallikrenin–kinin axis. These three systems appear to be intimately connected, forming a self-regulatory cascade that modulates renal perfusion, systemic blood pressure and sodium excretion. The relative importance of these systems is currently under investigation. Fig. 10.2 shows the interaction of the kallikrenin–kinin, RAS and prostaglandin systems.

The kidney is clearly not an organ which serves solely as a filter and waste disposal unit. The kidney is both the source and target tissue for a number of inter-related hormones which control functions as diverse as ion balance, plasma volume, vascular tone, blood pressure, erythrogenesis and calcium metabolism. We propose that the kidney should be considered an important part of the neuroendocrine axis.

Appendix

The appendix contains four tables which summarize the sites of synthesis and major metabolic effects of hormones referred to in earlier chapters.

Hormone	Chemical nature and site of synthesis		Homoeostatic blood concentration*	Major target tissues
INSULIN	Polypeptide mol. wt 5000 Pancreatic β-cells	= 51 amino acids	0.5–0.8 ng/ml (6–25 m U/L)	Liver, adipose, muscle
GLUCAGON	Polypeptide mol. wt 3485 Pancreatic α-cells	= 29 amino acids	0–50 pmol/L	Liver, adipose
GROWTH HORMONE	Polypeptide mol. wt 27 000 Anterior Pituitary	= 191 amino acids	0–11.5 m U/L	Liver, adipose, muscle
ADRENOCORTICOTROPHIN	Polypeptide mol. wt 4500 Anterior Pituitary	= 39 amino acids	6 a.m. 10–50 ng/L 6 p.m. 10 ng/L	Adrenal cortex
VASOPRESSIN	Oligopeptide mol. wt 1000 Posterior Pituitary	= 9 amino acids	0.4–0.8 ng/L (1–2 mU/L)	Kidney
OXYTOCIN	Oligopeptide mol. wt 1000 Posterior Pituitary	= 9 amino acids		Smooth muscle of uterus and mammary gland
PARATHORMONE	Polypeptide mol. wt 9500 Parathyroid	= 84 amino acids	10–55 ng/L	Kidney, bone
THYROTROPHIN	Polypeptide mol. wt 28 300 Anterior Pituitary	= amino acids	0.1–4.3 mU/L	Thyroid
CALCITONIN	Polypeptide mol. wt Thyroid 'C' cells	= 32 amino acids	100 ng/L (fasting)	Bone, kidney
THYROID HORMONE	Amino acid derivative Thyroid	T_3 = 651 (mol. wt) T_4 = 767 (mol. wt)	T4 53–135 nmol/L T3 0.9–2.5 nmol/L	Muscle, liver, kidney
PROLACTIN	Polypeptide mol. wt 22 000 Anterior Pituitary	= 199 amino acids	male < 400 mU/L female < 650 mU/L	Mammary gland, ovaries, testes, kidney, foetal lung
GLUCOCORTICOID	Steroid Adrenal cortex (zona glomerulosa)		Cortisol 9 a.m. 280–700 nmol/L	Muscle, liver, adipose
MINERALOCORTICOID	Steroid Adrenal cortex (zona fasciculata)		Aldosterone Adults 100–450 pmol/L	Kidney
CATECHOLAMINES	Amino acid derivatives chromaffin tissue, adrenal medulla		Adrenaline 0.02–0.04 ug/L Noradrenaline 0.2–0.4 ug/L	Cardiovascular system, muscle, adipose, pancreas (liver), thyroid, parathyroid, kidney

* Reference ranges are those given by the Department of Clinical Chemistry, City Hospital, Nottingham and are reproduced with the permission of Dr C.B. Marenah, Consultant Chemical Pathologist and Dr N. Lawson, Consultant Biochemist.

Table A2.   Some metabolic effects of insulin and glucagon

Insulin	Glucagon	Process	Tissue
↑		Glucose uptake	Muscle
↑ (both)	↓ (liver)	Glycogen synthesis	Muscle
↓ (both)	↑ (liver)	Glycogenolysis	Muscle
↓	↑	Gluconeogenesis	Liver
↑ (muscle)	↑ (liver)	Amino acid uptake	Muscle
↑		Protein synthesis	Muscle
↑	↓	Lipogenesis	Adipose
↓	↑	Lipolysis	Adipose
↓	↑	Ketogenesis	Liver

Table A3.   Major metabolic actions of cortisol on carbohydrate, protein and fat

Carbohydrate	↑ Gluconeogenesis
	↑ Peripheral antagonism to insulin
Protein	↑ Degradation ↓ synthesis in muscle
	↑ Concentration of circulating amino acids
	↑ Synthesis of gluconeogenic enzymes in liver
	↑ Ureogenesis
Fat	Hyperlipaemia; hypercholesterolaemia; Centripetal distribution of fat

Table A4.   Some metabolic effects of catecholamines

Tissue	Effect	Result
WHOLE BODY	↑ Thermogenesis	↑ metabolic rate
LIVER	↑ Glycogenolysis	↑ glucose output
	↑ Gluconeogenesis	
	↑ Ketogenesis	↑ ketone body output
	↑ K⁺ uptake	↑ maintains K⁺ homoeostasis
ADIPOSE TISSUE		
(White)	↑ Lipolysis	↑ blood FFA
(Brown)	↑ Lipolysis	↑ local thermogenesis
MUSCLE	↑ Glycogenolysis	↑ lactate output
	↓ Glucose uptake	↑ blood glucose
	↑ Ca²⁺ uptake	↑ contractile strength
	↑ K⁺ uptake	
KIDNEY	↑ Gluconeogenesis	↑ glucose and ammonia output
	↑ Free water clearance	↑ urine output
	↑ Na⁺ reabsorption	↑ ECF
	↑ Ca excretion	Hypercalciuria

Index